AT PEACE

AT PEACE

CHOOSING A GOOD DEATH
AFTER A LONG LIFE

Samuel Harrington, MD

GRAND CENTRAL
Life & Style

NEW YORK • BOSTON

Grand Central Life & Style
Hachette Book Group
1290 Avenue of the Americas, New York, NY 10104
grandcentrallifeandstyle.com
twitter.com/grandcentralpub

First edition: February 2018

Grand Central Life & Style is an imprint of Grand Central Publishing. The Grand Central Life & Style name and logo are trademarks of Hachette Book Group, Inc.

The publisher is not responsible for websites (or their content) that are not owned by the publisher.

The Hachette Speakers Bureau provides a wide range of authors for speaking events. To find out more, go to www.hachettespeakersbureau.com or call (866) 376-6591.

Library of Congress Cataloging-in-Publication Data

Names: Harrington, Samuel (Physician), author.
Title: At peace : choosing a good death after a long life / Samuel Harrington, MD.
Description: First edition. | New York : Grand Central Life & Style, 2018. | Includes bibliographical references and index.
Identifiers: LCCN 2017034568| ISBN 9781478917410 (hardcover) | ISBN 9781478923800 (audio downloadable) | ISBN 9781478917434 (ebook)
Subjects: LCSH: Terminal care—Popular works. | Terminally ill—Popular works. | Geriatrics—Popular works. | BISAC: SELF-HELP / Death, Grief, Bereavement. | SELF-HELP / Aging. | MEDICAL / Geriatrics.
Classification: LCC R726.8 .H365 2018 | DDC 616.02/9—dc23
LC record available at https://lccn.loc.gov/2017034568

ISBNs: 978-1-4789-1741-0 (hardcover), 978-1-4789-1743-4 (ebook)

Printed in the United States of America

LSC-C

10 9 8 7 6 5 4 3 2 1

I want to dedicate this book to my parents, who inspired it by living well and dying peacefully; my sisters, who worked together to make those transitions possible; and my wife, who encouraged me to reinvent myself after my medical career—an incomplete endeavor.

Author's Note

Most of the medical scenarios and examples are drawn from my professional experience with individual patients. Some examples are composites made from multiple patients; then they are introduced as "hypothetical" or "representative."

Where patients' names are used, they have been changed to protect their privacy.

This book does not intend to dispense specific medical or legal advice. It is written to inspire older patients and their families to view aging, disease, and dying through a personal lens that challenges the status quo of the medical establishment. In doing so, it raises awareness about medical and legal issues that affect end-of-life decision making. Medical decisions should be discussed with your physician. Legal decisions should be discussed with your lawyer.

Contents

Introduction   xi

Part One
Limits and Failures of American Medicine

Chapter 1: Good Death, Bad Death, Better Death?   3

Chapter 2: American Health Care: Failing the Elderly   12

Chapter 3: The Denial of Old Age: Immortal in America?   28

Chapter 4: The Median *Is* the Message   49

Part Two
Understanding Disease

Chapter 5: How Different Diseases Lead to Common
Causes of Death   63

Chapter 6: Deathbed Scenarios: How Does the End
Finally Arrive?   92

Chapter 7: Dad's Final Weeks   110

Chapter 8: How to Recognize a Terminal Diagnosis   119

Part Three
Practical Aspects of Planning for Death

Chapter 9: The Value of Your Prognosis   143

Chapter 10: The Hard Conversation   157

Chapter 11: Hospice Care   177

Chapter 12: Voluntary Refusal of Fluid and Food   196

Epilogue: Reflections and a Road Map   211

Abridged Chronology: Mom and Dad's Decline   224

Appendixes

Appendix I: Advance Directives   229

Appendix II: Dementia   245

Acknowledgments   255

Notes   257

Resource List   271

Index   275

About the Author   283

Introduction

Death is very likely the single best invention of life. Remembering that I'll be dead soon is the most important tool I've ever encountered to help me make the big decisions in life.

— Steve Jobs

The seeds for this book were planted almost a decade ago. I was sitting in my father's sunlit apartment overlooking the vast expanse of Lake Michigan. He was eighty-eight years old and the picture of health for his age. We were discussing treatment options for a ballooned blood vessel, an aortic aneurysm, in his abdomen. His internist had recommended a surgical consult, and three separate surgeons had recommended a standard operation to permanently repair it. I expressed concern that despite his appearance of good health, such a taxing abdominal operation and the associated prolonged recovery threatened to upset his independent lifestyle. Worried about the risk of rupture and wanting him to live long enough to meet his first great-grandchild, whose birth we expected in six months, I was promoting an alternative outpatient procedure: the insertion of a strengthening stent designed to reinforce the aneurysm for up to five years.

My father stunned me with a question that crystallized many ideas that I had been pondering over the last few years of my medical practice. "Why would I want to fix something that is going to carry me away the way I want to go?" he asked. Apparently he had the generally accurate impression that if his aneurysm ruptured, he could demand pain medication, decline emergency surgery, and be dead from internal bleeding within a few hours—a day or two at the most. His message was that he did not want a lingering death, and a ruptured aneurysm held an intellectual appeal for him in that regard.

More important, his question resonated on multiple, more complicated levels. First, it demonstrated a vision of his death that we, he and his family, could use to make future end-of-life decisions. Second, it demonstrated a willingness to gain knowledge about his ailments. Third, it indicated an acceptance that death was inevitable and that having a plan—a strategy—to manage it gave him some semblance of control. Finally, his question taught me to challenge the advice physicians, including me, reflexively give patients late in life.

Ultimately, my father had the outpatient procedure I advocated, and he met his great-granddaughter soon after her birth.

A year later, I was speaking with my older sister on the phone. She was preparing to visit our dad, and concerns about his health were weighing on her mind. She was bracing herself for her role as the oldest daughter. She was preparing herself to nurse him where necessary but more likely to organize his remaining time according to his frequently stated wishes to die at home and to do everything possible to avoid a nursing home placement. "You can't believe the wreckage in those places," he repeated. No excessive medical care for him, thank you very much. She would create an assisted living situation in his apartment. We would protect him as best we could.

Our mother had died three years earlier. We had thought our

father would wither and die. Contrary to our expectations, he soldiered on. But now, one year after his aneurysm treatment, his rugged independence was feeling threatened, and death was on his mind. Had he experienced a premonition? He wanted to visit with his daughter.

What if–type questions poured forth from her. Channeling his willingness to forego treatment if it meant a manageable death, I answered her.

"What if he has a stroke?" she asked.

"Call me," I replied.

"What if he gets pneumonia?"

"Call me."

"What if he falls?"

"If he is injured or in pain, call 911; otherwise, call me."

"What if I come in and find him dead in bed?"

"Wait until he is cold and blue, then call 911."

"Okay, I can do that."

Little did we know that he would live another five years.

———

This is a book about exit strategies. It is, indeed, another "end-of-life" book. It is not about making the end of life good. It is about making the end of life less bad. It is not about extending life. It is not even about extending "high quality" life. It is about avoiding a painful dying process and futile medical care. It is not a philosophical treatise about what makes life worth living. It is simply a practical look at declining health, old age, progressive debility, and practical choices that people can make to minimize the likelihood of the unconsidered death and to maximize the likelihood of a "better" death.

This book is not about physician-assisted suicide, medical aid in dying, or "death with dignity," although I will mention them in chapter 12. It is about developing a vision for a natural death—a death caused by disease or old age but not influenced by the violence of excessive medical technology.

This book is not going to dwell on ethical arguments for or against end-of-life choices, but I will state the ethical position responsible physicians take regarding life-sustaining treatments. It is the duty of the physician to sustain life and relieve suffering. When the performance of one responsibility conflicts with the other, the physician must defer to the patient's wishes.

This book is not about control. I understand that to suggest that we can control our deaths is simplistic and borders on falsehood. All deaths represent a loss of control. We can lose control to the natural history of old age and disease, or we can give up control to doctors and their therapeutic interventions. We can never keep complete control.

Finally, this book is about acceptance. That acceptance is not limited to the emotional acceptance described by Elisabeth Kübler-Ross as the fifth stage of loss and grief in her 1969 book *On Death and Dying*.[1] That emotional component is part of it, but I also encourage acceptance based on knowledge and understanding.

The goal of this book is to outline disease processes or trajectories and to emphasize choices that minimize the chances of a medicalized death and maximize the chances of a better death.

By disease trajectory, I mean the average course of illness for a given diagnosis. By medicalized death, I mean the state of a semi-conscious patient in an ICU or nursing home who is subjected to medical treatments beyond their direct wishes or beyond common sense. Therefore, the restated goal of this book is to use the knowledge of disease trajectories to choose a point in the disease process at which one considers stopping aggressive treatment and recognizes that palliative treatment is likely to offer a better outcome.

———

Steve Jobs's quote that "Death is very likely the single best invention of life" sounds brave. It has been used for purposes of inspiration by at least one hospice organization.[2] It sounds as if he really understood that all things must end. It sounds as if he accepted death. However, this is only because the quote is taken out of context; both the context of the speech and the context of his life.

The quotation was included in his commencement speech delivered to the graduating class at Stanford University in 2005. He had recently been diagnosed with a rare form of pancreatic cancer but lived six more years, dying in 2011. "Remembering that I will die soon" informed his business decisions specifically. That knowledge did not inform his medical decisions. "Steve never passively accepted end of life, nor did he have palliative care," wrote his biographer, Walter Isaacson.[3]

The reason I am dwelling on this is that Jobs's arrogance reminds me of my own. I recognize that it is arrogant to suggest how people should die. It is arrogant to suggest that people can control their fate. But many elderly people die while suffering excessive medical care that could have been limited if they had considered the alternative to fighting until the end.

Just a hint of philosophic perspective follows here. What makes humans forget that we are not immune to death? What makes every generation think that it will be the first generation to live much longer and much better? What makes each of us deny our illnesses and assume that we will "beat" old age or a terminal illness?

Perhaps it is the immutable will to live. Perhaps it is this century's conflation of a religious eternal life with a secular immortality. Perhaps it is a coping mechanism for an overwhelming fear of death. Perhaps it is the centuries-old confusion of science and magical thinking.

Each generation has its "immortalists." Charlatans who sell the promise of eternal youth are everywhere. Scientists who allow the goals of their restorative or life-prolonging research to be described as "just around the corner" (instead of decades away) abound.

The current generation is obsessed with youth because youth "sells." Diets, additives, exercise programs, and mental exercises all deny the inevitable. The beauty and fitness of our aging (but cosmetically enhanced) celebrities leap off the Photoshopped covers of glossy magazines with the promise of endless well-being.

This book is about recognizing that death is universal and will be so until this book is long out of print. This book is about recognizing the limitations of modern medicine in extending life expectancy; it is about the high physical and emotional cost of attempting to extend one's life in the face of the inevitable; and it is about recognizing when to face death on your own terms and not someone else's.

This book is aimed at several types of readers. First and foremost, it is written to inform the elderly and chronically ill patient who is in need of guidance at the end of life. Second, it is written to inform the families and caregivers of the elderly and chronically ill who, as agents of a patient, might be responsible for making difficult end-of-life decisions. Third, it is written for anyone who can look far enough ahead to know that death will arrive and to see that preparing for it in personal terms is better than leaving it completely to chance or in the hands of overly aggressive doctors.

Finally, it is not written for younger patients battling premature cancers or other illnesses. Such patients might take away some lessons or ideas, but I do not presume to have easy answers for their prematurely tragic circumstances. I have written it with the goal that each type of reader can see the important points from their own perspective.

The bulk of the book is devoted to informing patients and

empowering them to make informed decisions. At some point in the process of decision-making, acceptance must occur. Some readers will think that acceptance is another way of saying, "Give up." I am not saying that. At the point of acceptance, I am saying, "Become aggressively passive." Seize control of the decisions. Stop letting the physicians make the decisions. Review their recommendations but do not accept every one.

I understand that aggressive passivity sounds like giving up, but it is not. It is taking control of the one thing you can control: your care. It is a step taken at the point in life when you see a loss of control over everyday activities and bodily functions. It is the step to be taken when you see (with the help of this book) that you can no longer control your disease, and by fighting it you allow it to control you. Recognizing that once intensive medical treatment is initiated, its momentum and outcomes are largely out of your control, and declining such treatment puts you back in charge.

———

This book is broadly divided into three sections.

The first section of the book defines "a better death" and debunks aspects of the American health care system. The endless optimism of the politicians, the false hope of the advertisers, and the exaggerated promises of providers demand a reality check. Emotionally and spiritually, people have a powerful will to live, but intellectually we deny the inevitable. One of the reasons we expect to live forever is this false hope of a cure just around the corner and this false sense that American medicine is beating the odds.

The second third of the book describes disease trajectory and deathbed scenarios. In his classic work *How We Die*, Sherwin Nuland described multiple illnesses and death scenes. Using different clinical scenarios, his elegant prose grimly and honestly detailed how the body deteriorates and life ends in the randomness and messiness of debility, disease, and death. The second section of this book dovetails with that concept and expands on it to show that, despite the differences of every clinical situation, there are also some commonalities. I describe the concepts of acute and chronic illnesses. I describe the course of illness for the six chronic diseases that cause the majority of adult deaths.

I will show that despite the randomness of illness there are recognizable patterns. Despite the unpredictability of the final act, a patient suffering from a chronic illness can take action and assert some influence on the outcome.

The final section of the book deals with practical aspects of the difficult conversations that result in responsible decisions. There are chapters on prognosis, end-of-life conversations, hospice care, and the voluntary refusal of fluid and food. A summary and a road map follow.

Finally, there is an appendix that takes a look at the details of advance directives and the unique challenges of dementia.

————

My father lived five years after the procedure to reinforce his aneurysm. Three of those years were good years, but two of them were not. The good years were characterized by continued activity and independence. The bad years were characterized by progressive weakness, physical limitations, and the dependence on others that my father had hoped to avoid. But by posing his original question about the wisdom of repairing his aneurysm my father informed his family and caregivers about his vision of a natural death. That vision informed all of his subsequent medical decision-making.

It is my hope that you, the reader, will enjoy the book. Doing so will help you gain a healthy skepticism of the American health care system, its marketing excesses, exaggerated promises, and the motives of its providers. I hope you will also get insight into disease trajectories, better decisions, and, ideally, a vision that you can share with your family.

Combining the understanding of disease trajectories, an appreciation for the process of natural death, and skepticism of a system designed to treat excessively with practical end-of-life decisions will help patients have a better chance at a better death.

Part One

LIMITS AND FAILURES
OF AMERICAN
MEDICINE

Chapter One

Good Death, Bad Death, Better Death?

> [1] To every thing there is a season, and a time to every purpose under the heaven:
> [2] A time to be born, and a time to die; a time to plant, and a time to pluck up that which is planted;
>
> —Ecclesiastes 3, King James Version

M Y FATHER DIED quietly, at home. He was one month and one day shy of his ninety-fourth birthday. His mantra was "I have lived too long." Indeed, I agreed with him until he was gone and then it was, instantaneously, not long enough.

He died a "good death." He died a natural death. And, because of his slow decline, each of his children had every opportunity to visit, reflect, reminisce, and review the various ledgers of our lives with him.

I am the second of four children. I have three sisters. We each had a role throughout his life. We each had a role during his long decline. My oldest sister managed the business and household side of his decline. I was in charge of the medical advice. My middle sister, the earliest to retire, hosted him most frequently and extensively while he was still able to travel. My youngest sister, still working and with the most restricted schedule, kept him grounded and inspired.

My mother died a good death, too.

My mother, the bedrock of our childhood, had died of lung cancer seven and a half years earlier. She also died at home, at peace, and quietly. I gave medical advice to her and to my father, but I did not control the decisions. Although my mother was subtly demented she made her will known, and they made decisions together.

My mother was fading and physically weak by the time she was eighty years old. She had weathered multiple illnesses throughout her life. I was not privy to most of them and was not asked to opine about them. She was a stoic, phlegmatic New Englander who did not dwell on her diseases, their causes, their cures, or their detritus. The scar on her neck, the multiple stress fractures, the orthopedic shoes, the misshapen breast prosthesis and, nearer the end, the memory lapses told the story of multiple conditions: a parathyroid adenoma, osteoporosis, degenerative arthritis, breast cancer, and mild dementia.

Ten months before she died, she was diagnosed with pneumonia while she and my father were making their winter pilgrimage to my middle sister's home in California. She was much weaker and frailer than my father. He remained a robust eighty-six-year-old man who exercised daily, took French lessons, played the piano, and remained active in the geriatric community while caring for her. She was still cooking simple things and organizing their apartment's domestic needs, but she used a "traveling chair" for long excursions or when transiting through airports.

As is so common at her age, the pneumonia was an infection superimposed on a lung cancer.[1] I do not remember the details of their return home to Milwaukee, the CT scans or the biopsy site, but I do remember the resultant diagnosis of stage IV, non–small cell carcinoma of the lung.

I also remember my first conversation with her, face to face, the next month. I explained to her that the median survival of her cancer was ten months after diagnosis.[2] "That means, Mom, that if there were a hundred patients with the same diagnosis here in your apartment, first, it would be very crowded and second, half of them will have died by October. We just don't know which half." I made the mental note to myself that at her age and with her frailty she was more likely to die before the median than after.

She looked at me and asked, "Are you telling me that I am going to die?"

"Yes, Mom, but I don't know when."

My father sat quietly. He was clearly in anguish. They had been the closest of companions for the last twenty years since his retirement. These were probably the best years of their marriage. But it was clear to him that she was not a fighter. He was the dominant member of the pair. He was physically stronger and, at this stage in their lives, he was emotionally stronger. In some couples, the stronger member will fight to survive to support the weaker, but it is rare for the weaker to try to prolong his or her life for the stronger. It was understood that Mom was not going to suffer aggressive treatment so that she could be there a bit longer for him.

After studying treatment options, their schedule, and their lifestyle, Mom and Dad made plans based on doing less treatment, rather than more. Those decisions flowed naturally. It was clear that Dad would care for her and was aiming at a quiet death at home.

Mom chose low-dose chemotherapy with one goal in mind; she wanted to see her oldest grandchild get married four months later. It was the first wedding in that generation, and Mom was prepared to fight to see it. Instinctively, she set that goal. Just as naturally, she recognized her grim prognosis, and she knew when to stop fighting. Her career in nursing had taught her to be realistic and to aim for the best possible day.

Prior to the trip for the May wedding, she was admitted to home hospice care and acquired a Do Not Resuscitate (DNR) status from her doctors. Exhibiting rare, raw emotion, Dad did not allow her to wear her DNR bracelet, preferring to carry it in his wallet.

After the wedding, she discontinued chemotherapy and passed the summer at home. In September, she asked, "Am I getting stronger?" No one told her the truth, which was "No."

A few weeks later, my mother did die quietly at home. She was in hospice care but not bed-bound yet. She was still taking meals at the table, tea and cocktails in the living room, and sleeping in her own bed. To that degree, her death was unexpected but a blessing because she did not suffer the painful complications of lung cancer.

My sisters and I thought that there was a real chance that my father would give up and die shortly thereafter. He did shrink socially. He did fade physically. Then he rebounded.

About five years before his death it became clear that Dad needed help around the apartment. The staff of their residential hotel did some weekly cleaning chores, and he cobbled together a schedule of simple breakfasts, luncheon sandwiches, restaurant meals, leftovers, and the occasional dinner guest. But laundry, dish washing, humidifiers, plant care, and other tasks, began to loom large. We hired a young woman to help out for a few hours per day. Dad's desire to "wake up dead" became a recurrent mantra. My older sister and I had several conversations on the subject.

Despite the absence of a terminal illness, Dad acquired his own DNR status. We counseled each other, and advised his young helper that if he was found unresponsive (but comfortable) some morning, she should call me before calling 911.

As our expectation that he would die within a year faded, we realized that his decline would be unbearably long. We had presumed that he would give up and die before the weakness of old age set in. But he did not give up, and weakness did set in.

It was a slower death than Mom's, but they were both "good" deaths. My parents asserted what they would not do medically and took control. They were not in pain. They both visited with family. They trusted their caretakers. They understood their illnesses.

Although the vision of their deathbeds changed over time, they firmly held that the vision would not include hospitalization or nursing home residence.

They did not trade a bit of high-quality life for low-quality existence.

THE MEDICALIZATION OF DEATH

How do you want to die? Do you want to suffer? Do you want your last conscious sensations to be the chest compressions of an emergency medical technician (EMT) separating your sternum from your ribs? Do you want your last sight to be the specter of a tracheal intubation blade approaching your mouth followed immediately thereafter by the insertion of a tube into your lungs? Do you want people rushing to stab large-bore needles into your neck and groin to access big, reliable veins?

Do you want to die in an ICU, on a ventilator, unconscious, unrecognizably bloated, oozing from sores and pores, every orifice violated with a tube, and unable to communicate with family and friends? This is not hyperbole. This is what saving people from near death looks like. Cardiopulmonary resuscitation (CPR) is much more brutal and much less effective than people are led to believe. When a patient is young and has a reversible condition this situation is disturbing, but acceptable. When the patient is old, infirm, or suffering from a terminal illness, this situation is cruel and reflects poor judgment.

That is because the chance of surviving to discharge from the hospital is 0 to 8 percent.[3] And the chance of returning home neurologically intact is less than that.

Alternatively, do you want to die warehoused in a nursing home, surrounded by elders who are infirm and incontinent; fighting bedsores and begging for a diaper change; being spoon fed or tube fed; and being aided by well-intentioned, but understaffed and underpaid, nursing services?

These images depict the "medicalization" of an institutionalized death that has dominated medical treatment and patient expectations for the last fifty years and has come to define the new normal of prolonging life at all cost. Some people, following the lead of Groucho Marx, "intend to live forever, or die trying." For younger patients with prematurely terminal diagnoses, this is an understandable treatment pathway. For elderly patients, those who have lived beyond their "average life expectancy," this is a mistake.[4] Those people are likely to die in one of the scenarios depicted in the previous paragraphs. I respect that many people choose to place themselves in a situation where they are likely to die (in agony) in an ambulance, emergency room, or ICU. Others choose repetitive interventions for bladder infections, pneumonias, heart failure, and so on, with the result that they die slowly in the comparative isolation of a nursing home. These are the elderly who want to fight to the end and want to be remembered for having done so. If they understand the price they will pay for their decisions, then I say, good luck to them, for they risk losing the opportunity to say goodbye, make amends, and find peace painlessly.

Most people who do not want to fight endlessly envision dying quickly. Having survived the grief following my mother's death, my father wanted to "wake up dead." It was his shorthand for dying in his sleep. He had expressed this desire for several years. Unfortunately, this result is enjoyed by only a small fraction of the population. It is a chance event that involves no control on our part. Practically speaking, the technological advances of the last few decades have decreased the size of heart attacks and strokes. These advances, along with improved trauma care, respiratory care, and less invasive surgical techniques, have reduced the absolute number of acute deaths. The effect is that those of us who do not die suddenly or unexpectedly will die older, later in life, with progressive disability and diminished faculties. "Old age" will be our terminal diagnosis, and living longer than desired is likely to be our punishment for lack of planning.

A BETTER DEATH

Or would you consider something else? This book is about resisting the momentum to treat and recognizing the moment to care.

Most people want to avoid futile and painful treatment. Most elderly people express a preference to die at home but cannot afford that if it means a prolonged decline requiring round-the-clock assistance. Therefore, nursing homes—which are best utilized as a way station for rehabilitation and temporary skilled nursing needs—become long-term residences. Unfortunately, when entering a nursing home or assisted living facility or arrangement without effective advance directives, the patient becomes dependent on the care of the organization. As the disability of old age progresses and physical independence is lost, the resident falls into the trap of the perpetual treatment that the system is organized to deliver with the risk that the residence becomes a warehouse of bedridden bodies.

If, while still cogent, you put in place the decision-making paperwork that would allow for early hospice registration and restrictions on nutritional support, hospitalization, and aggressive medical treatment, then a long, uncomfortable, lonely decline in a nursing home can be avoided.

Should you so desire, many people can afford to return home for their final days or weeks if they foresee the nursing home as a way station and if, with the help of hospice nurse guidance, they recognize the last phase of life, the stage of "active dying" (to be discussed later) that heralds the last days.

I prefer to think that people, unconstrained by a personal belief (cultural or religious) that they should suffer as long as possible, would prefer this different course. I want to promote planning that will maximize the possibility that one can pass away surrounded by friends and family, with minimal suffering, uninterrupted by ineffective medical interventions, at home (if desired or possible) and at peace.

GOOD, BETTER, BEST

I cannot define a "good death" in a way that will satisfy every reader. Each person must come to his or her own definition of that. Such a definition is highly individual and changeable over the course of an illness. But when it has been studied, a good death includes control, comfort, closure, affirmation, trust, understanding, and communication.[5] In my experience as a practicing physician, these attributes are usually inconsistent with an institutionalized death associated with aggressive medical treatments.

It might be easier to start with a definition or example of the "best death." My vision of that is to die in one's sleep, naturally, spontaneously, and shortly after a large family gathering involving good food, various tributes, a review of a life well spent, and expressions of appreciation for one's family and their accomplishments, at an age that equals, or exceeds, the average life expectancy. Hoping for more is unrealistic and risky.

If we cannot guarantee that the "best" death will occur, then we must work toward a "better" death, a death that is less bad than the hospitalized process and less bad than an institutionalized existence.

Therefore, my "better" death will have to be initiated a step back from "waking up dead" and a step before calling 911. It will have to include a conscious recognition that you have had enough treatment. It will mean that you understand the limits of American medicine and that you do not want to risk inviting a medical intervention that might become self-perpetuating. Unwilling to call 911 and unable to count on dying in your sleep, you will need to institute a plan that will maximize your influence and minimize ineffective or unwanted medical intervention.

As I will make clear in subsequent chapters, this strategy is not "death with dignity" or assisted suicide. This strategy is a combination of medical passivity (informed by medical knowledge), hospice care, explicit advance directives, and a vision of the deathbed that reflects your personal preferences. This strategy involves the recognition and acceptance of the inevitable and, most important, an image of the possible.

My parents died naturally and with dignity because they had such a vision and could foresee the process.

Things to Remember/Things to Consider

- Consider your concept of a good death.
- Think about the level of medical intervention you want. Outline your goals and expectations.
- Communicate your goals and wishes to your friends and family while you are still able.
- Remember, aggressive treatment to the very end results in futile and painful therapies.
- Look for opportunities to review less aggressive options.

Chapter Two

American Health Care: Failing the Elderly

When medicine became a business, we lost our moral compass.
—Steven Nissan, MD, *Escape Fire*

THE UNITED STATES has the costliest health care system in the world. It spends almost twice as much per capita as the next costliest country, yet it has comparatively poor outcomes. The fact that the American public does not understand or believe this is the result of the advertising and lobbying campaigns of one of the most powerful commercial and political alliances ever organized. In 2015, US health care spending represented 17.8 percent of the gross domestic product.[1]

In a special article published in 1980, Arnold Relman, editor of the *New England Journal of Medicine*, popularized the phrase "the medical-industrial complex" to detail these powerful forces. A takeoff on President Eisenhower's concept that the military-industrial complex was driving our defense posture in the 1950s, Relman's point was that the medical-industrial complex was driving health care expenditures while blinding doctors and patients to the true principles of medical practice. Pharmaceutical companies and medical device companies have been funding research and medical education at all levels, including medical school, continuing medical education, and the dissemination of medical knowledge to providers and consumers. From 1960 to the present day, profit-seeking companies and their shareholders have driven the American health care system by spurring the commercialization of care and blinding providers to conflicts of interest.[2] These same companies have convinced consumers to expect excessive medical care, leading American patients to believe that a cure for whatever ails them is just around the corner while generally overlooking the compassionate, supportive, and thoughtful care the elderly patient really needs.

The lesson here for aging patients, their caregivers, their family, their friends, and their agents is that untempered hopefulness requires a slow, thoughtful reality check. Elderly patients—and here I mean patients over the age of sixty-five and suffering a chronic illness or people over the age of the average life expectancy for their demographic—should try to understand that they are not missing out on a miracle cure despite the societal hyperbole to the contrary. The rate of increase in the average life expectancy has slowed; and there are no cures for the most common chronic illnesses.

Most of the medical optimism Americans enjoy is based on exaggerated promises. If an elderly patient thinks they can "win the lottery," they are more likely to struggle on. If they believe that fixing one more joint or one heart valve will reverse the ravages of old age they will try for that winning ticket, and by doing so they are likely to pay the medicalized price for it. If they think that a politician's promise to deliver on personal cancer therapy will happen in their lifetime, they will hang on against all common sense. They will seek treatment that is likely to be futile, resulting in unnecessary pain and suffering.

THE PROBLEM WITH A SYSTEM
LIKE MEDICARE

From the patient perspective, Medicare has been a very successful health care insurance payment system—more efficient and user-friendly than the commercial insurance industry. However, over the last three decades, the routine decrease in government reimbursements has changed the providers' perspective on Medicare patients.

Initially, Medicare was created as a safety net for elderly citizens, and it proved to be a gold mine for fee-for-service physicians. Medicare patients were valued because the government paid handsome fees and the older population had plenty of diseases to treat. Since the 1990s, when reimbursements decreased, the perspective on elder care has changed. Now, the American health care industry treats the elderly as a commodity. To maintain their income stream, primary providers spend less time with elderly patients, and in the name of efficiency procedure-oriented specialists such as gastroenterologists, cardiologists, and surgeons treat Medicare patients as widgets, rushing them through an assembly line of procedures without adequate consideration or consultation.

In areas where younger, higher paying patients exist, the elderly are spurned. Where money can be made by overtreatment, they are churned, i.e., run through the system. Where reimbursement is low, the elderly receive short shrift or are ignored.

AT THE INTERFACE OF TECHNOLOGY AND
AGING: WHERE HIGH-TECH TREATMENTS
MEET ASSEMBLY-LINE CARE

The failure of modern medicine is not only about the hype, the PR, and the political posturing that lead to overblown promises of fabulous treatments. It is also about omissions contained in incomplete consultations about technological advances in cancer chemotherapy, immunotherapy, joint replacement surgery, and new cardiac devices.

One of the reasons for our extraordinarily high expenditures is the overproduction of resources (hospitals, surgery centers, laboratories, radiologic equipment) that allow for immediate access but demand utilization. There is no need to wait for a hip replacement in the United States. We have plenty of orthopedic specialists, too many MRI machines, too many operating rooms, and too many physical therapy units. For all these same reasons, there is no need to wait for cardiac surgery. In terms of convenience for elective and semi-elective procedures, the United States is the best, especially if the procedure is lucrative.

A subtle example of the "churning" of elderly consumers is the development of a specialized service—a product line or service line, in the vernacular of a hospital's business development administrators. In my former hospital, we developed joint replacement surgery as one such product line to attract patients. Other hospitals might emphasize a service line in cardiology, gastroenterology, or oncology, for example.

The creation of these service lines involves the development of therapeutic protocols, the hiring of supplemental support personnel (physicians, nurses, social workers, physical therapists), and some degree of promotion or advertising. It has the intent of focusing expertise, developing the efficiencies of systemized treatments, and benefitting by the economies of scale. Unfortunately, promoting a product line or "center of excellence" raises expectations, instills an assembly-line mentality, turns some physicians into salespeople, and reduces unwary patients into consumers, thus distorting a traditional doctor–patient relationship.

To be fair, done well, assembly-line care does reduce complications and increase quality when patient selection is tightly controlled. And extra "hospitalist" care for complicated patients improves medical outcomes.[3] But there are several unintended consequences that occur. First, just as safer highway engineering inspires drivers to increase their speed, better outcomes tempt physicians to treat older and weaker patients. Second, by supplying more hospitalist care to deal with the medical complications, the medical or surgical specialist is less invested in deselecting patients who are likely to have limited benefit or who have a higher risk of complications. And third, it takes less time to plug an overeager patient into a system of care than to advise them that system was not built with their individual needs in mind.

MEDICAL CONSEQUENCES OF ASSEMBLY-LINE CARE

The result of assembly-line care is a subset of patients undergoing procedures following incomplete or one-sided consultations. In the case of my hospital's service line—orthopedics—there were patients receiving elective joint replacements who should have been advised, "I can replace your hip, but surgery comes with prohibitive risks at your age." Or "Replacing this hip will put more strain on your other joints and you will still be restricted by your weak back." Or "I know you feel restricted by this bad joint, but adjusting to that restriction is more sensible than risking surgery."

Over the years, I saw increasing numbers of unrealistically optimistic patients who underwent orthopedic surgery, cardiac procedures, gastrointestinal procedures (including some done by me), or aggressive chemotherapy because they were led to believe that quality of life could only improve and we, physicians, knew that we could get them through. Too little time was spent during the associated consultations describing those patients who did poorly despite surgery or those patients who did well enough without surgery. These practices contributed to a downstream accumulation of elderly patients with minimal benefit, post-op complications, prolonged hospitalizations, and nursing home placements.

And most patients were not advised of what awaits every elderly patient admitted to a hospital for any reason: some degree of further, overall deterioration.

When elderly patients have complicated elective (or semi-elective) surgery, it is guaranteed that they will be exposed to large quantities of antibiotics and narcotics. They are guaranteed to have their usual medication regimes disrupted. They are very likely to receive blood thinners to prevent clots from bed rest. They are likely to suffer a general physical decline from forced inactivity.

During my career, I witnessed too many complications that would not have occurred in the absence of elective surgery and other aggressive treatments on elderly people. I saw dozens of gastric and colonic hemorrhages as a result of non-steroidal anti-inflammatory drugs (NSAIDs) and blood thinners. I saw scores of patients intubated for surgery and then reduced to bed rest because of general weakness and pneumonia. I saw countless patients with paralyzed bowels, the consequence of excessive narcotics.

This is not so much the result of bad medical practice as it is the result of a system that is not focused on the holistic needs of the elderly. The misaligned interest of the technically skilled surgeon, the hospital-based internists used to dealing with medical crises, the hospital administration, and the assembly-line mentality that fixes one joint, one valve, or one manifestation of cancer among many frequently overlooks the aging patient as a whole.

The assembly-line mind-set should be avoided during the consultation phase and the patient selection process. It should start only at the execution phase, when the patient is prepared to roll through the doors to the operating room.

CHRONIC DISEASE, ACUTE CURES, OVEREMPHASIZED SCREENING PROGRAMS

There are other structural weaknesses in the American health care system.

The American health care system is well designed to treat acute problems like a broken wrist, appendicitis, pneumonia, or an initial heart attack or stroke. It has the technology and wherewithal to reverse most acute illnesses successfully and rapidly. But curing pneumonia does not cure any underlying chronic illness, be it lung disease, heart failure, dementia, stroke, diabetes, or cancer.

People over sixty-five should recognize that the diseases that will define their later years are likely to be chronic diseases set in motion years, if not decades, earlier. Three realities follow this understanding: First, treating acute complications of chronic disease does not "cure" the patient but prolongs the chronic process. Second, more frequent treatments of more complicated scenarios in more debilitated patients lead to more risk, more complications, and accelerated debility. And third, screening tests (like colonoscopy or mammography) for inactive diseases in the chronically ill or frail elderly patient will not prolong life, because that patient is likely to die from their current and active illness.

In short, our system has not focused on the long-term care of the chronically ill, most of whom are elderly. Whereas acute illnesses have cures, chronic illnesses have treatments that must be organized and managed. That type of management requires a health care system that is integrated, supportive, and communicative. The medical marketplace has yet to find a profit-making formula to create such a system. So we fall back on short-term treatments of the complications of chronic diseases.

We all understand that preventing disease is preferable to an expensive treatment. We forget, however, that real disease prevention relies on lifestyle choices that avoid toxic chemicals, bad habits, and too many calories. Instead, we are encouraged to assume that if we find a disease early, it can be cured or curtailed. The result is that health care providers in a for-profit system learn that screening for illness is a more lucrative practice than effective counseling on healthy lifestyles.

Screening even for common illnesses, when looked at objectively, is not simple.[4] Witness the controversies surrounding screening mammography and prostate cancer blood tests. But screening for low-probability illness in the general population is a strategy of dubious benefit. When it comes to screening for low-probability illnesses in the chronically ill or elderly, it is a strategy that can be cruelly counterproductive. For example, a colonoscopy performed to reduce the risk of colon cancer in an elderly person without symptoms can lead to one of several possible outcomes. Most will be normal, so it will have been a waste of time. Some will remove a colon polyp that is unlikely to shorten the patient's life expectancy, so it, too, will have been a waste of time. Very rarely such a screening colonoscopy will reveal an unsuspected cancer. This will prematurely set in motion the surgery and subsequent treatments that foretell the patient's demise.

There is one other possible outcome: A complication could occur. For example, many elderly will be unable to finish the prep to get an adequate exam, resulting in a wasted exam. On occasion, frail patients will pass out and hurt themselves during the preparation. Rarely, but with measurable frequency, something more serious happens.

CONFRONTING MY RECOGNITION OF MEDICINE'S LIMITS

I started my career in gastroenterology devoted to eradicating colon cancer. I planned to do the most thorough and comprehensive colonoscopies possible. I committed myself to the idea that none of my patients would get that disease on my watch. The sequence and transition of benign polyps growing and turning into colon cancer seemed to be the perfect example of a disease progression that could be interrupted.

When I first went into practice, the recommendation for a screening colonoscopy was to perform it at age fifty and every five years thereafter. If a polyp was discovered, a surveillance exam would be repeated in one year and every three years thereafter. Thirty years later the screening interval had been extended to ten years and the surveillance interval to five years. Still, patients came in much more regularly than that. New scopes with better optics helped find smaller and subtler polyps. Here the pace of new technology outpaced the development of new guidelines. Research supported by the scope manufacturing industry defined new types of polyps that were presumed to represent threats not included in standard surveillance recommendations. As a result, practitioners were educated to believe that patients required more frequent follow-up exams.[5]

By the end of my career, we could find polyps that were less than a millimeter in diameter, and magnification allowed us to see blood cells circulating within them. Yet the mortality for colon cancer did not significantly decline.

In my personal practice I found and removed countless precancerous polyps. I found many cancers deep within the wall of the colon, including those that were too small to have started with a visible polyp—defying the widely held view that all colon cancers can be prevented by removing all polyps. I can think of at least one patient who developed a large cancer between recommended screening exams. Did I miss it with the last screening exam? Did it grow faster than average? Fortunately, he survived surgery and did not require radiation or chemotherapy.

As time passed and more exceptions and complications occurred and as more guidelines failed to clarify our practices, I realized that surveillance colonoscopies were only addressing one pathway in the formation of colon cancer. And, despite more numerous and more increasingly expensive exams, we were only reducing, not eradicating, colon cancer. As a result, I lost confidence in much of the system and its promises.

One of my most memorable complications occurred after an apparently healthy seventy-eight-year-old woman was referred to me for a screening exam. She had never acquiesced to a colonoscopy before, but her internist finally convinced her. The conventional wisdom was that a single initial exam, no matter at what age, was likely to be beneficial. The conventional wisdom did not factor in extra scar tissue (adhesions) between her spleen and her colon. The exam tore her spleen, and she nearly bled to death. A surgeon saved her life and my composure.

The complication of splenic rupture occurs once in 100,000 colonoscopies. It is not operator dependent. It was not due to an error on my part. Rather, it is preordained by a congenital attachment of the spleen to the colon. The fragile spleen is subsequently torn as the colon is routinely straightened during the exam. "You can't play baseball without breaking some knuckles," is how some of my colleagues remember their complications. I responded with despair at the damage the exam had caused. I remember watching a surgical colleague stop a life-threatening hemorrhage. I also saw a previously active patient return home debilitated from days in bed and weeks in the hospital. All this was caused by a screening exam performed for a purely theoretical benefit.

FAILURE TO CONTROL THE MANAGEMENT OF ANTIBIOTICS

Though my father suffered no irreversible disaster as a result of the American health care system, he did have a brush with an antibiotic-related complication when he was eighty-nine years old—a complication that was the result of decades of overuse of antibiotics by American physicians. Disaster was averted only because his problem fell within my field of expertise. But his experience exemplified how aggressive treatment of what appeared to be a trivial problem can go awry.

Late one spring, five years before he died, my father was aiming to attend a memorial service for his deceased sister-in-law and the wedding of his second grandson. Both these events were scheduled within a few weeks of each other in Massachusetts. He could still travel by himself, but he was at the point of counting his steps, in terms of distance, and stairs, in terms of heights. He was using a wheelchair in the airport and a cane for walking. We were also helping him seek handicapped rooms in hotels and handicapped parking on the streets.

During the run-up to these travel plans, he had a deformed toe amputated. The hope was that if his foot functioned better, then his walking would improve. The surgery was scheduled weeks before the memorial service so that he could be completely healed and back in walking shoes before the trip. Standard procedure dictated that he take a pre-op dose of antibiotics for skin contaminants and a post-op oral course of antibiotics to prevent the most common foot infections. Even though this surgery could have been performed with an antiseptic wash and without systemic antibiotics, "prophylactic" antibiotics have become the norm because the average patient does not take good enough care of a foot wound following surgery.[6]

One week before travel, he developed loose stools. Within a day or two, to his horror, he had soiled himself. That is when I was notified of his problem, for there is nothing like an episode of incontinence to crystalize one's concerns about dependency. Advised of that symptom, I knew he had an infection with *Clostridia difficile*. *C. diff.* is a species of bacteria that naturally exists in 3 to 6 percent of the healthy population. Typically, it causes no disease, because it is suppressed by the presence of multiple other organisms. But, if an otherwise healthy carrier takes an antibiotic, that person is at a grave risk of killing the good bacteria and releasing the *C. diff.* from its suppressed state. Such an overgrowth releases toxins into the colon that cause diarrhea and kill colon cells, a disease known as *Clostridia difficile* colitis or antibiotic associated colitis (AAC). If the colon becomes sufficiently damaged, the process can lead to gangrene of the colon, and this is usually fatal. Once a rare disease, the relentless overuse of antibiotics has resulted in an increase of AAC. At the end of my clinical career, *C. diff.* infection was by far the most common cause of diarrhea I saw in my practice.

After a brief discussion, I prescribed vancomycin, an antibiotic antidote specific to this infection. We had only seventy-two hours until the memorial service, and it took that long for the treatment to work in most people.

Dad got better. He attended the memorial service. He enjoyed the wedding. And he learned a lesson.

When he needed additional foot surgery, the doctor treated him with topical antiseptics. Subsequent dental surgery was treated without antibiotics at all. Though his experience with a complication of systemically overused antibiotics resulted in added personal cost, inconvenience, and mild embarrassment, it could have been much worse. In 2011, 29,000 people died of AAC. Most of them were elderly.

THE MOMENTUM TO TREAT

The momentum to treat in America is unmatched around the globe or throughout history. As a result, we spend twice as much on medical care as the next most expensive country. A very large percentage of that money is spent in the last six months of life. There are multiple forces behind this momentum.

In her book *Ordinary Medicine*, Sharon Kaufman explains how

Medicare has contributed to the growth industry of eldercare.[7] While Medicare began as the arbiter of what is reimbursable, in the minds of providers and patients it has become the adjudicator of what is appropriate care. The conclusion being that if a new treatment is available, it might be appropriate, but if it is reimbursable from Medicare, then it must be appropriate.

What else fuels the momentum to treat? American exceptionalism, for one. This is an ingrained feeling that the United States and its citizens are not only different but are the best, have the best, do the best, and deserve the best. As a result, most Americans pridefully believe that American medicine is the best in the world. These Americans are dead wrong. Compared with other developed countries, American medicine is unexceptional except in terms of cost, convenience, and self-promotion. In terms of things that matter—such as life expectancy, infant mortality, or quality of life after sixty-five—the United States ranks in the lower third of developed countries, sometimes dead last. Yet American exceptionalism inspires acquiescence in patients, which makes resistance to treatment almost unpatriotic. When coupled with the profit-over-principle mentality of providers, this momentum to treat contributes to the medicalization of death.

Additionally, the momentum to treat is powered by the competition between health care systems. Unfortunately, systems such as the Cleveland Clinic, the Mayo Clinic, and Johns Hopkins do not compete in terms of doing the most ethical or compassionate work but in terms of doing the most technologically advanced and financially rewarding work. This is exemplified by a conversation I had with a transplant cardiologist from the Tufts University medical system. He acknowledged the ethical questions raised by performing so many left ventricular assist device (LVAD) insertions on elderly patients in an effort to support them for a possible future heart transplant.[8] In the next breath he said with pride that their annual use of LVADs was up 80 percent, and they were now doing more transplants than their nearby competition, the Harvard system.

Add media manipulation to the mix of Medicare reimbursement, American exceptionalism, and competitive systems, and we have created a recipe for disaster for the aging population.

Only two countries, New Zealand and the United States, allow direct-to-consumer pharmaceutical advertising. This advertising has led to increased consumption and unrealistic expectations. In turn, this leads to inappropriate treatments.[9]

Three years before leaving my practice, I met an elderly patient who developed late-onset ulcerative colitis. Vigorous for an octogenarian, she was a comparatively active socialite who found that the bloody diarrhea and near incontinence that her disease caused was unacceptable. I was sympathetic, and we were both disappointed by her response to standard therapy. Through advertisements, my patient was aware of infliximab (brand name Remicade), an infusion that altered the immune system. I was hesitant to start such a treatment because of her age (there were limited studies performed in elderly patients and there were many warnings against its use in that population), but she and her family were insistent. We sought the advice of an expert in inflammatory bowel disease. My hope was that the second opinion would support my recommendation that the patient avoid this sophisticated treatment and adjust to her new, reduced circumstances. There was always the chance for a spontaneous remission.

Unfortunately, the physician providing the second opinion promoted and initiated the new treatment. In the end, it proved easier, less time consuming, and more profitable for the expert simply to plug the patient into their assembly line than to explain repeatedly why she should consider resisting that system. Shortly after the first infusion, the patient reported a dramatic improvement in her bowel symptoms. Two weeks later she was admitted to the ICU with double pneumonia caused by an organism released by her weakened immune system. Still in the ICU, she died two weeks after that.

This patient remains a case in point. At $4,000 per infusion of infliximab, she was unlikely to undertake it without Medicare reimbursement. She believed the advertisements that exaggerated the benefits and minimized the risks. She did not believe that her life could or should be limited by illness at her advanced age. Instead, she died prematurely and suffered a medicalized death.

A VISION OF LIVING TO THE END RATHER THAN FIGHTING TO THE END

Courtesy of the medical-industrial complex, we as a nation think that we are on the brink of a series of cures for the great scourges of our time. This, coupled with our ability to delay death by treating acute illnesses, tempts people to seek treatment that ultimately becomes futile and risks a drawn-out decline and a painful death with too much medical intervention. Ironically, the longer we live as a population, the larger the problem of chronic diseases becomes.

Technological advances in the treatment of heart failure (pacemakers, defibrillators, heart pumps, and heart valves) prolong lives, but they do so with an emotional toll placed on those not comfortable with an unnatural mechanical dependence.

We are losing the war on Alzheimer's, as a tsunami of baby boomers approaches old age. And, having made much progress, we are now stalemated in the war on cancer. Fortunately, progress will continue on all fronts—witness the paradigm shift to "individualized cancer care" based on identifying DNA segments in different tumors—but gains will be incremental, costs will be exponential, and unforeseeable complications will develop.

So what is the alternative to endless treatments of acute events superimposed on progressive chronic illness? What is the alternative to ceding control to overly aggressive physicians? The alternative is to develop a vision of where the chronic illness is going and what a better death might look like. This vision recognizes that aging and dying are natural processes that require management. By resisting the momentum to treat, you avoid ineffective and painful treatment. By managing your care, you take control back from the medical establishment. By having a vision of aging and dying, you can develop a vision of living purposefully in comparative comfort rather than fighting futilely while enduring prolonged suffering.

Things to Remember/Things to Consider

- American health care is driven by conflicting imperatives to care for patients and to make a profit.
- Assembly-line care improves efficiency and quality but can overlook compassion.
- Remember, every hospitalization, including elective treatments, risks progressive weakness and unintended consequences. Be skeptical.
- Certain medications and treatments can be high risk for little gain, like aggressive chemotherapy for advanced cancer or immunomodulation therapy in elderly patients.
- The momentum to treat can often obscure the absence of a cure and delay comfort care.

Chapter Three

The Denial of Old Age: Immortal in America?

But our machines have now been running seventy or eighty years, and we must expect that, worn as they are, here a pivot, there a wheel, now a pinion, next a spring, will be giving way; and however we may tinker them up for a while, all will at length surcease motion.

—Thomas Jefferson

THE MOMENTUM TO treat is propelled by forces other than those described in the last chapter. Indeed, the will to live is perhaps the foundation of the momentum to treat. Hope and its alter ego, denial, form the core of the will to live, and I will discuss them in detail in chapter 10. But now I want to focus on a blend of internal and external forces that fuse our intrinsic hope with our acquired overexpectation.

At the intersection of American exceptionalism and media manipulation lies a uniquely American persona filled with hopefulness, optimism, anticipation, and expectation. Courtesy of our society's emphasis on youth, celebrity, and consumerism coupled with the successful marketing of medical advances, health care products, and political promises, much of this optimism is based on overstatements.

In a provocative essay published in *The Atlantic* in October 2014, Ezekiel J. Emanuel coined the phrase and named this character "the American immortal."[1] He describes this individual as obsessed with exercise, mental puzzles, diets (juices, nuts, berries, protein), and vitamins (antioxidants, etc.). Their practices are the result of the fusion of American exceptionalism and a belief in the concept that by living a longer healthy life, one is likely to die more suddenly, with less disability and dependence. In his essay entitled "Why I Hope to Die at 75," Emanuel details why obsession with living longer is misguided and why the actions of immortalists are frequently counterproductive and potentially self-destructive.

In fact, Emanuel does not want to die at age seventy-five (the title was an editor's choice) but he does make a strong argument for refusing non-palliative medical care after that age. His arguments are reasonable, but they include many value judgments (e.g., living too long transforms how people remember us; by age seventy-five most of our creativity is gone; living too long burdens our children) that one can quibble with. He also promotes several concepts that are underappreciated, such as dying at an old age is a loss but not a tragedy; some people believe that mindlessly extending life is purposeless; and living too long is associated with loss and grief.

I disagree with the arbitrary age cutoff, but do agree with his other conclusions. My takeaway lesson is that if we don't assert control over the end of our lives some other, well-intentioned family member or provider will. More important, the processes that have created the American immortal are driving the momentum to treat.

Immortalists have lived in every generation and every culture, but the American "baby boomer" generation represents a large, uniquely entitled, and overly optimistic group. The leading edge of that demographic bulge is approaching age seventy-three, just a few years shy of the average life expectancy. The trailing edge has long been influencing the decisions of their aged parents.

TO DIE YOUNG, LATE IN LIFE: A STATISTICAL CONCEPT OR A LIFESTYLE GOAL

In defining the American immortal, Emanuel invokes the concept of the "compression of morbidity." This scientific concept, that we are living longer healthier lives and dying quickly with less disability, was introduced by James Fries in 1980.[2]

Fries wrote that we entered the twentieth century with an average life expectancy of forty-seven years during an era of infectious disease when tuberculosis was the number one killer. By the late twentieth century reductions in mortality of 99 percent by these infectious diseases and other advances in medicine had pushed the average life expectancy to seventy-three (seventy for men and seventy-seven for women). Now the average life expectancy is about seventy-nine years.

In addition, and very importantly, he convincingly argues that the length of human life is biologically fixed and states that "statistics suggest that under ideal societal conditions, mean age at death is not far from eighty-five years." Combining the increase in average life expectancy with a fixed limit to absolute life expectancy, he concludes that this results in the "rectangularization of the survival curve" with more people living longer, dying faster at a more advanced age, and suffering shorter periods of disability.

1. The Increasingly Rectangular Survival Curve

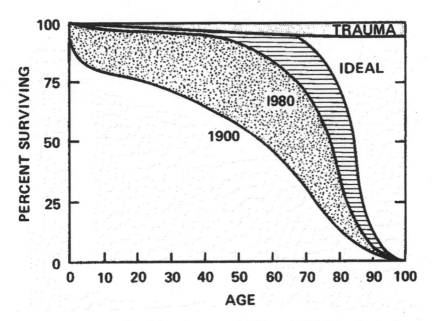

Figure 1. Fries's original graph from the New England Journal of Medicine *showing the rectangularization of the survival curve. According to this, 50 percent of the population dies by age fifty-five in 1900 and by age seventy-eight in 1980. With permission from the* NEJM.

This is the scientific basis and statistical explanation that the excessively health conscious intuit as proof that their lifestyle obsessions will help them fulfill their doctor's tongue-in-cheek encouragement to "die young, as late in life as possible."[3] It is the scientific theory reinforcing the assumption of the American immortal that by consciously living a healthy life (as defined by the media promulgating lifestyles and products) one will live well until they die. If correct, then no end-of-life planning is required. A problem with this conclusion is that if we live healthy lives into old age and die while physically fit, that death might seem chronologically appropriate but is physiologically premature.

2. Compression of Morbidity

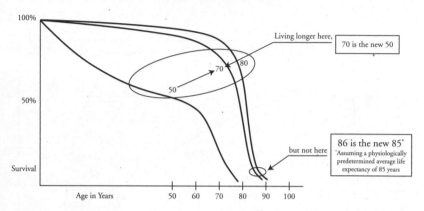

Figure 2. The author's reinterpretation of Fries's graph showing that 70 is the new 50 and 86 is the new 85.

But what this graph really shows, as depicted in figure 2, is that the maximum improvement in health and survival occurred between ages fifty and seventy. There is comparatively little change between the ages of seventy-five and ninety. Or, put differently, if seventy is the new fifty, then eighty-six is the new eighty-five, and those of us lucky enough to survive into our eighties will still have to deal with the same survival rate (and period of disability) as decades ago.

DISABLED YEARS AFTER SIXTY-FIVE

How many years of life expectancy after sixty-five are healthy years and how many are disabled years is an important subject for researchers and policy makers. The current conclusion is that the average life expectancy is increasing about a year per decade and disabled years after sixty-five are decreasing, albeit by about two months per decade. This type of information may be used to determine changes in eligibility for Social Security and Medicare or other demographic questions related to government policy. But from the patient perspective, whether disabled years after sixty-five are increasing a bit or decreasing a bit is academic.

What is important to note is that if a person reaches the age of sixty-five in reasonable health they have an average life expectancy of almost nineteen years. Of those nineteen years, ten and a half are likely to be healthy years and eight and a half are likely to be disabled years. Practically speaking, these numbers have been steady for decades. Equally important to note is that one year before their death, 80 percent of Americans are living lives complicated by disability.[4, 5]

This latter fact should comfort us by helping us recognize that we are not dying prematurely. But the former fact should discomfit us. By focusing on the concept of "dying young, late in life" and embracing the slight trend toward fewer disabled years after sixty-five, Americans who think themselves immortal consciously refuse to entertain a vision of aging and dying. They ignore the impending disability of old age and subconsciously conclude that they can go on forever.

Although the current population of the oldest patients is more likely to be made up of members of the "greatest generation" and have had more exposure to alcohol and cigarettes, with the exception of potentially less chronic lung disease, the baby boomers are not likely to redefine the deterioration of aging and the chronic diseases that carry us away. Contrary to what the very health conscious believe, the body of scientific evidence shows that antioxidants do not prevent cancer; exercise does not guarantee the absence of heart disease; sudoku does not prevent dementia; and stress reduction does not create a flawless and impenetrable immune system.

If we are lucky enough to get old, we should be prepared for some disability.

HEALTHY LIFESTYLES OFFER NO GUARANTEES

We can all name examples of nutritionists who died of cancer (Adele Davis) or long distance runners who died of heart disease (Jim Fixx). We all know that mental exercises can improve function and mental acuteness at any given time, but they do not alter the fundamental course of dementia. Above and beyond the irrefutable fact that everybody dies of something, it is clear that targeted activities reduce the risk of a disease process primarily by being the opposite of behaviors that cause that disease. Targeted behaviors do not change the inevitability of getting a chronic illness if one lives long enough, and targeted behaviors do not eradicate a specific disease.

The behaviors of the overly health conscious and the decisions they make have the potential to be personally damaging in a variety of ways. Concrete examples include exposure to unregulated compounds in vitamins and supplements as well as unhealthy practices such as detox programs and fad diets. Excessive exercise may lead to premature bone and joint deterioration (degenerative joint disease or arthritis). Indirectly, and more importantly, the mind-set that healthy practices will indefinitely forestall death permeates their thinking and obstructs the development of a vision of the inevitable.

Blending the exaggerated promise of diet and supplements with a gullible population of patients promotes the misconception of an easy fix. About fifteen years ago I participated in a panel discussion at my former hospital. A nutritionist, a colonoscopist (myself), a surgeon, and an oncologist presented their perspectives on the prevention, detection, excision, and treatment of colon cancer.

After the presentation, questions were asked and answered. The audience, almost all older than sixty-five and many colon cancer patients among them, directed most of their questions to the nutritionist. A typical question was, "How many blueberries do I have to eat per day to prevent colon cancer?" Of course, if blueberries prevented colon cancer the disease would have been eradicated by now. The questions implied a wishful naïveté that belied the effect of the processes already in motion in the intestines of the audience participants. I am sympathetic to the desire for an easy fix. Unfortunately, some blueberries will not reverse the cumulative effect of decades of the American diet, and few wanted to hear that.

We can all agree that unhealthy lifestyles shorten life expectancy. Every cigarette reduces one's life expectancy by seven to ten minutes, for example. But there is little evidence that a specific lifestyle reliably enhances life expectancy beyond the average. Healthy lifestyles, encouraging moderation in all things, should be promoted with the expectation that they will decrease the chances of premature death, but will, therefore, increase the likelihood of death by old age or a chronic illness. Lifestyle zealots need to remove their blinders. They need a plan, too. If your strategy is to die late in life, then you should acknowledge that you will be old and will need a strategy to die better.

Of course, the American immortalist is a caricature of a personality type. But that exaggeration embodies a truth about the influence of overexpectation behind the momentum to treat. More important, a belief in the promises of our system resides hidden in the breast of the majority of patients. That overexpectation feeds the hope and denial that seek endless treatments. These treatments prolong the dying process; expand the duration of debility; increase the risk of painful medicalization; and, ultimately, prove futile.

MEDICAL CARE AFTER SEVENTY-FIVE

The average life expectancy for the American male is about seventy-seven and for the American female about eighty-two. It is worth

noting that these numbers vary based on other demographic factors such as race, wealth, and education. But, as stated before, if one
reaches sixty-five in good health, one can look forward to an average
of almost nineteen more years. Conversely, one must consider that
reaching sixty-five in the presence of a chronic illness will lower one's
life expectancy accordingly. In either group (after age sixty-five but
with a chronic illness and after age eighty even if appearing healthy)
aggressive medical care should be thought through carefully. After one
has reached the average life expectancy, the balance between the risk
and benefit of aggressive medical treatments shifts. The potential to do
harm rises in the elderly or chronically ill and the long-term benefit, by
definition, declines.

Several professional memories pop to mind when thinking of American immortalists in my practice. One patient was a successful lobbyist and consultant. He described himself as an avid off-trail skier. His
skiing career ended following multiple back surgeries and joint replacements. Condemned to a walker or wheelchair, his functional status
was destined to deteriorate. Independent of his obsession with skiing,
his stubborn reliance on his idea of a healthy diet to control his chronic
diverticulitis blinded him to ignore my advice for elective surgery. Emergency surgery resulted in a colostomy and accelerated debility.

When my elderly patients reported, with pride, that they were still
enjoying tennis, biking, skiing, or boating, I wanted to say, "Hey, why
not take it down a notch and start water aerobics?" But what I said was,
"Still playing tennis—what are you playing, quadruples? Seriously, be
careful, if you fall and break something it will cause a real setback."

Several of my patients lived to be more than a hundred. My oldest
died at 107. He made frequent visits for a colon that kept twisting on
itself, a problem that I could easily, albeit temporarily, correct with a
short colonoscopy.[6] Too old for definitive surgery and "blessed" with
good genes, he lived on and on. What I did not envy about his existence

is that he had lost much of his dignity. The nurses and techs in my hospital and his nursing home treated him like a pet, a cute anomaly. But it is easier to be patronizing than honest: "Mr. Cameron, you are a hundred and seven years old; how much longer do you want to go on?" "We need a plan for when this easy fix isn't easy or stops working."

One very devoted patient died at one hundred. He did not share the misguided optimism of the classic immortalist; he was simply irrepressible. He had fought through multiple illnesses. He ignored my recommendation to refuse a new heart valve at ninety-six. I think he fought through two years of post-op rehabilitation just to prove me wrong. I am glad he did, but there were times that even he was not so sure he had made the right choice.

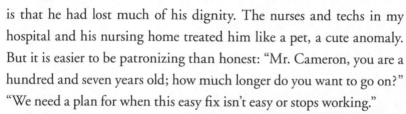

A STRATEGY TO DIE BETTER

A strategy to die better is an important concept in our personal efforts to take control of the last phase of our life. The focus should be the willingness to see that after one has achieved the average life expectancy, it is the rare person who can expect to retain long-term youth. By the time you have started to dwindle, you have outlived the theoretical benefit of the compression of morbidity. Fighting hard against a chronic disease may seem heroic, but fighting too hard is likely to result in a medicalized death such as that of my elderly colitis patient (see chapter 2).

If you find yourself or your loved one in the state of decline that frequently visits people with a chronic illness and advanced age or simple debility at a very advanced age, please consider any intervention with real promise for benefit. But also consider the real possibility of a complication and plan accordingly. Discuss in advance such a complication and plan to establish a line in the sand: not Emanuel's arbitrary seventy-fifth birthday, but a combination of disease, weakness, and functional status beyond which you will allow only palliative care.

My father, who died one month shy of ninety-four, began to disengage from active medical care around age ninety. After that time he sought only selective medical help, and he gradually peeled off his physicians and all active medical care. He stopped all medications three months before his death, having entered a home hospice three months before that. I am convinced that by becoming passive on medical care he not only prolonged the quality of his life but, unintentionally, its duration. Most important, he avoided painful, ineffective medical treatments.

MY FATHER'S STORY

My father enjoyed an extremely vigorous performance status until the age of eighty-nine. He walked without a cane. He drove neighbors to the Jewish Community Center for water aerobics. He could walk endlessly, but paid little attention to fitness goals. He was not a Fitbit type. He managed his affairs. He dealt with chores around the apartment. But age was creeping up on him.

About five years before his death, Dad slipped on the floor in his kitchen. It was an eye-opening experience. He cracked his head, without losing consciousness, and bruised his lower back. Fortunately, my youngest sister was visiting; otherwise my siblings and I might never have known. She called the rest of us to report, and the four of us consulted.

We discussed the physical reason behind the fall. It turns out that Dad was losing sensation in his feet. A peripheral neuropathy, caused by age and alcohol consumption, had robbed him of the ability to feel where his feet were in space and when, exactly, they touched the floor. That sensory loss conspired with a slick linoleum floor and a pair of wool socks to produce the fall and the realization for us all that his veneer of good health was cracking. It crystallized the understanding that he was not yet "old" but that he was aging.

Within the month, my sisters had organized some domestic help to check in on him, prepare light meals, do laundry, and water the plants. His first employee was a young art student in need of supplemental income. She proved to be the most important hire of his retirement. She stayed with him to the end, replicating the providential relationships that bless so many end-of-life scenarios.

Of course, after my mother's death the family began discussing assisted living options and potential nursing home choices. Dad was adamant that he preferred cobbling together a team to create an assisted living scenario in his own apartment to the alternative of moving into a local facility or moving close to one of his children. "I can't afford assisted living facilities," he would argue disingenuously.

He was even more adamant that he did not want to move to a nursing home and that he would do everything possible to avoid that eventuality.

It was clear, however, that that fall was the beginning of his journey into the disability of old age. He needed physical therapy to strengthen the back and leg weakness caused by the fall. He started using a cane. Years later he moved to a walker, a transport chair, and a wheelchair. Familiar with counting steps and stairways when caring for my mother, he began to apply those principles to his daily life. He began avoiding restaurants, theaters, and stores with difficult access issues. His world began to shrink. He became less independent. It was painful to watch.

With respect to personal independence, one scene in particular remains vivid in my mind. I escorted my father to the airport after what proved to be his last trip to Maine. We checked his bag, and an attendant arrived with a wheelchair to escort him through security and take him to the gate. Dad put the tip of his cane on the footrests and crossed his hands over the handle. He shrank back into the chair.

The attendant asked if I wanted to accompany them through security and wait until the plane boarded. "Sure, thank you," I responded.

"No, I will be fine," my father insisted. He did not want to further share his reduced state with me. He was grieving for his independence and recognizing his diminished performance status for what it was: the beginning of being old.

As the next few years passed, we discussed how every setback required more prolonged and less successful rehabilitation. One course of physical therapy resulted in a hamstring tear that was frustratingly hard to diagnose and that led to weeks of pain. Dad started to refuse physical therapy sometime after that experience. I told him, as I had told so many of my patients, that Henry "Red" Allen said it best in his 1930s blues song, "You Might Get Better But You'll Never Get Well."

"Don't quote the blues to me," he responded. "The tune you should reference is 'You've Been a Good Old Wagon, Daddy, but You Done Broke Down.'"

Thomas Jefferson was seventy-one when he wrote this chapter's opening quotation to John Adams, indicating that he recognized the disability of aging.

My father recognized it when he was ninety-one.

THE DISABILITY OF OLD AGE

How does one define disability? How does one quantify it? These are worth considering in making calculations about the course of a disease and the process of aging. In the context of this discussion the general understanding of disability must be expanded to include the effect of aging. In this regard I regularly use the term "debility" to describe the physical (or mental) weakness that old age imparts.

Disability comes in many forms. When we see a space reserved for a handicapped person, we might envision that someone using a wheelchair or walker will occupy it. But many disabilities acquired with old age are less obvious—though equally limiting—and include deafness, visual deterioration, loss of muscle mass, loss of dexterity, nerve damage, diminished exercise tolerance because of poor circulation, and loss of dental soundness. Debility, specifically, is the weakness of illness or aging that ultimately saps our independence and renders us wheelchair dependent or bed-bound. It is not subject to improvement with treatment or rehabilitation.

The acquired disability of the elderly need not be dramatic to be important. Swapping out dress shoes for slippers with Velcro straps does not define debility, but it is a manifestation of decreased manual dexterity. Functional problems with feet, joints, vision, hearing, and even dental decay can be major quality-of-life issues and ultimately lead to decreased performance status. The progressive loss of performance status is a means to understanding aging. Performance status can be monitored and quantified, including distances walked, stairs climbed, or time passed sitting without fatigue. These can be measured, and personal observations, compared over time, can demonstrate the rate of decline.

Institutions and regulatory agencies use activities of daily living (ADLs) and instrumental activities of daily living (IADLs) to quantify levels of disability and need in people with disease-wrought limitations (e.g., paralysis after a stroke) and the progressive weakness of aging. ADLs include the self-care actions of bathing, dressing, eating, toileting, and getting in and out of a bed or chair.[7] IADLs define the ability to be independent and include preparing meals, food shopping, managing money, using the phone, and doing light housework. As one loses one IADL after another, one needs more assistance and assistants. As one loses one ADL after another, one needs more caretaking. Lose them all, and one needs a detailed care plan or a way out.[8]

QUALITY OF LIFE AFTER SIXTY-FIVE: WHEN DO YOU BECOME OLD?

Of course, we must not confuse the disability of a young person with a long life expectancy (a spinal injury after a motor vehicle accident, for example) with the disabling weakness of a person at an advanced age. In the former scenario, where rehabilitation offers potential improvement, accommodating to the disability can lead to good quality of life. In the latter scenario, where rehabilitation has limited benefit, accommodation leads to increased dependency, accelerated frailty, and progressive grief.

"Quality years after age sixty-five" is a moveable target and subject to endless definitional debate. In developed countries we expect good quality years after age sixty-five. Each individual reader will have to decide for him- or herself what constitutes good quality. If you can afford to read this book, by virtue of education and income, you probably have a good quality of existence when compared to less fortunate Americans. That does not mean that it will last or that it was the action of American medicine that got you to this place. If you have arrived at an advanced age, the American health care system might have influenced that outcome, but it is more likely that the good fortune of healthy genes, an education, a good socio-economic status, and the absence of a few harmful lifestyle practices were more important. Wherever you are on the spectrum of quality of life and independent living, eventually, that system and your genes will fail you. If you do not die acutely, you are likely to die disabled. How much debility and how you choose to cope with it is the question.

How do we recognize when we are not aging, but have become elderly? Is it when we need help cooking and cleaning? Probably not. Is it when we need help bathing or toileting ourselves? Is it when we cannot raise ourselves up from the floor after a slip or a fall? Is it when, even with the help of our spouse, we cannot get up? These should not only be thought of as inconveniences that require work-arounds but as milestones from which there is no turning back.[9]

When a person becomes disabled by age or disease, it does not matter whether they lived the life of a couch potato or a marathon runner. Disease and disability progress with age. The statistical reality of the compression curve might hold true for the decades between ages fifty and seventy, but that is of no comfort to the elderly person dwindling at home or in a nursing home. If we don't die young, we will die disabled.

More recently, Fries, the proponent of the compression of morbidity theory, agrees that we are now in an era of chronic disease (atherosclerosis, neoplasia, emphysema, diabetes, cirrhosis, and degenerative arthritis) and that a third era is in our future. He advises that this will be the era of senescence, "when the aging process itself, independent of specific disease, will constitute a major burden of illness for the United States."[10]

Whether from illness or senescence, the disability of old age is the accumulation of insults resulting in the progressive inability to care for ourselves.

Suffering from debility, my father thought that he died too slowly. It was three years from the time that he recognized his need for household assistance because of reduced performance status. One of those was still a good year, but two of them were not. My mother died more quickly, but not too quickly. She lived nine months after recognizing her terminal illness. This gave plenty of time to organize visits and prepare our goodbyes. She was spared a prolonged trial of bed-bound decline. Perhaps her comparatively sudden death was from a blood clot, a disturbance of her heart rhythm, or another bladder infection, unbound. In any event, the suddenness of her death, after a ten-month illness, was a small mercy.

Why a few people like my mother die suddenly enough—but not too suddenly—and so many people dwindle much longer is a mystery to some but not to me. I am sure that if in her case we had searched for a potential blood clot, an irregular pulse, or a bladder infection we would have found something to briefly delay the inevitable. But we would have put her at risk of futile treatment and prevented a good death.

Why my father survived to dwindle, despite having disconnected himself from medical treatment and engaged himself only with nursing care, remains unclear to me. It was his fate to die slowly.

It is a comfort to me that they both died at home, comparatively peacefully, and naturally—as a result of their disease and without excessive medical intervention.

MORE CARE OR LESS CARE FOR THE ELDERLY?

Some would argue that more care for the elderly is better. They are sicker. They are weaker. We must fine-tune their care. We must examine them more closely.

A group of my colleagues made the bulk of their income by doing comprehensive annual physical exams. The yearly physical exam was part of the foundation of medical care when I began my practice. Since the 1990s it has been discredited as beneficial, but has lost little traction in practice. Studies show that the annual physical and its associated tests inflate cost and do not reduce morbidity and mortality. This fact is lost on the general public and ignored by those physicians performing "executive physicals."

Here is an example of how an annual physical combined with unnecessary (and, therefore, excessive) testing does harm, or at best, no good. Several years before leaving practice, I met a charming eighty-year-old woman, who lived with her equally charming, but more debilitated, sister. At the time of her annual physical exam, her diligent internist found her to have a slightly low blood count and a trace of blood in her stool. The low level of her blood count is a common, usually harmless, finding in the elderly. The trace of blood is usually a false positive. However, her internist referred her with the expectation that I would proceed with scope tests of her colon and stomach to exclude a potentially serious disease. The internist described her as very "vibrant," a coded request that I do as much as possible and not let her die of a gastrointestinal malignancy on his watch. The two sisters and I had a long discussion. I noted that they were very engaged, but both were very weak and frail with multiple functional limitations.

I talked the patient out of a colonoscopy. She had undergone such an exam by another practitioner within the last ten years and had probably maximized her (statistical) benefit at that point. I feared that the preparation would be very stressful and probably suboptimal. I also argued that if she was anemic from colon cancer it was probably too late and that the treatment for such a cancer (segmental colon resection and chemotherapy) would do her in.

We settled on an upper endoscopy to rule out benign blood-losing lesions and hoped that we did not find an unsuspected gastric malignancy. Unfortunately for her, I found a medium-size, flat, and benign growth on the inner curve of her duodenum (small intestine). Biopsies proved it to have pre-cancer potential. My bias, which I explained to her as both my professional opinion and a biased opinion, was to leave well enough alone. The lesion was at risk to grow and bleed, but it was a small risk. Theoretically, it could be used to explain the evidence of blood in the stool and some blood loss anemia. To manage it aggressively (that means to cut it out) would have required surgery (too aggressive at her age) or serial endoscopies to remove it piecemeal (the current standard of care). Each endoscopy would carry the small but cumulative risk of bleeding, perforation, anesthesia, and other complications. Given her age it probably would best be managed through benign neglect, and I told her, "If you were my mother, I would recommend doing nothing. Of course, if things did not work out as I predicted, then my mother would forgive me."

A triangulated conversation with the referring physician resulted in a second opinion with an aggressive academic endoscopist. The patient underwent serial endoscopies, and ultimately the lesion was removed without serious complication, although the frequent outpatient trips put stress on her sister and ended when the sister fell in the hospital and fractured her pelvis. They had learned a lesson and wisely refused the recommendations of the academic endoscopist for regular follow-up examinations to monitor for a possible recurrence.

It is clear that the only one who definitely benefitted from this treatment plan was the other endoscopist.

As I matured as a gastroenterologist, devoted to preventing colon cancer where it was useful to do so, I began to see that most doctors and patients envisioned no end to the usefulness of screening exams and associated testing. When to start screening and when to end screening are fundamental questions that medical science should be refining and redefining on a regular basis, but practitioners and patients resist any limitations. It was instinctively clear to me that some age existed after which screening did more harm than good.

In the geographic area within which I practiced there were several academic institutions. One aired multiple radio ads about screening colonoscopies saving lives. They also had an annual educational meeting at which they promoted their use of technology. Their well-established position on the radio airwaves and academic meetings was that colon cancer occurred at all ages and that there was no clear end point to the benefit of colonoscopies. The companies producing endoscopic technology and equipment subsidized the research

supporting this school of thought. This institution accepted all com-
ers and seemed to churn the geriatric population through colonoscopy
after colonoscopy.

But a more humane school of thought was growing. It held that
after a certain age (yet to be exactly determined) the presence of
advanced age and other illnesses indicated that a patient was so much
more likely to die of something other than a future colon cancer that a
preemptive exam was not justifiable.

During the last five years of my practice I was regularly turning
people away who were referred for a screening colonoscopy. I advised
them that a preemptive exam was unlikely to help them and might
harm them.[11] The vast majority of patients left the office saying,
"Thanks, Doc, I like that advice. I will call you if I have a symptom."

ARBITRARY DECISIONS VERSUS A VISION OR A PLAN

It is hard to do, but the pressure to treat should often be resisted. I
advised my patient and her sister against treatment that offered no
measurable, only theoretical, benefit. Yet her sister, her internist, and
a second consultant moved the agenda. "The momentum of medicine
and family means we will almost invariably get it [a test or treatment],"
wrote Dr. Emanuel.

In defiance of medical momentum, he wrote that he would not
have a screening colonoscopy after the age of sixty-five and that he
would decline cancer therapy, pacemakers, heart surgery, dialysis, and
even antibiotics after age seventy-five. But the real lesson of his essay
is not to decline medical treatment at an arbitrary age. The real lesson
is that he was thinking about these treatments at all and would not
accept them arbitrarily.

I enjoyed seeing my elderly optimist before and after his heart valve replacement at age ninety-six. I will never forget the day that he left the office, then leaned back in. Speaking across the waiting room to my medical assistant, he blasted, "Tell Dr. Harrington that I feel rampant!" It was an odd turn of phrase to describe his zest for life, and it prompted all the other patients to perk up and ask what I had done for him.

But, prior to that, when he chose to proceed with his heart surgery against my advice, he did not proceed blindly. We had a long pre-operative discussion about what to do and what not to do in the event of a complication. He had a vision, and we worked out a plan. I am glad there was no complication, because even with the best plan, when dealing with an aggressive treating doctor, like the heart surgeon, it can be difficult to back away. Surgeons don't want to compromise their statistics. But having no plan and no limits practically guarantees excessive treatment and increases the risks of a hospitalized death.

Things to Remember/Things to Consider

- Remember you are mortal, not immortal.
- Keep in mind that, on average, if you are lucky enough to live past the age of seventy-five, you are likely to have to cope with eight years of variable disability.
- Consider the occasional inventory of your age, diagnoses, disability milestones, and performance status.
- Understand that with age the risk of treatment increases and the benefit decreases.
- Consider a combination of disease, debility, and functional status beyond which you will not seek aggressive care.
- Do not look for potential problems with screening tests; address active illnesses purposefully.

Chapter Four

The Median *Is* the Message

Science continues to be a channel for magic—the belief that for the human will, empowered by knowledge, nothing is impossible. This confusion of science and magic is not an ailment of a kind that has a remedy. It goes with modern life. Death is a provocation to this way of living, because it makes a boundary beyond which the will cannot go.
—John Gray, *The Immortalization Commission*

M Y FATHER AND I talked about the median survival of an illness on two occasions. The first was when we three (my father, my mother, and I) discussed my mother's lung cancer diagnosis. The second conversation occurred some years later when discussing his abdominal aortic aneurysm. Both my parents understood that the median survival of ten months for lung cancer or the median time to rupture of six months for his aneurysm did not mean that death would personally visit them at that exact moment but that it would have visited half of all people diagnosed with the same conditions, quite possibly including them.

My father did not focus on his diseases as something to be treated, fixed, or cured. Instead, he focused on them as problems with which he had to deal. My father was considering the option of ignoring his aneurysm and using the potential rupture as a way to die quickly, a death he viewed as preferable to dwindling or lingering. He was not really giving up, but he was ready to stop fighting every condition and to accept what came naturally. Because his first great-grandchild was due in six months, my sisters and I talked him out of that position.

Years before that, a patient, described by his referring physician as "cantankerous and difficult," taught me a lot about the process of aging and a vision of dying. Alfred D. came to me to discuss colon cancer screening options. A retired electrical engineer, he lived quietly and comfortably in a pricey condo. He was overweight from drinking and short of breath from smoking, and he was not going to give up either vice.

"Doc, I am going to die of smoking or drinking—or maybe a heart attack. Until then, I am not going to change."

He refused my every suggestion to screen him for colon cancer, including a simple rectal exam ("Don't go there, Doc"), but he did transfer his general care to my office, presumably because I harangued him less than his original internist. Then one day he started bleeding from his rectum. Not part of his plan to die from smoking or drinking, he did allow a full evaluation including the rectal exam and colonoscopy that, if performed years before, might have prevented the rectal cancer that we now found so easily.

Professionally embarrassed for not having pushed him harder to perform the screening tests, I apologized. "Doc, I brought this on myself," he replied, and accepted full responsibility for his decisions. To minimize the need for radiation or chemotherapy, Alfred chose an extensive surgical resection and a colostomy (the bag on the side).[1] He never complained and he never looked back.

He remained a cantankerous curmudgeon. I remained his unaggressive internist. He continued to smoke and drink. When heart and lung disease made it too difficult for his wife to care for him, we signed him into a hospice bed in a nursing home, and he died quietly a few months later at the age of eighty-seven.

When we first met, I thought his decision making was driven exclusively by the pathology of his addictions. His response to his colon cancer taught me otherwise. Alfred foresaw his death by lung disease. He was stubborn but honest and self-aware. His cancer surgery informed him that he did not want to be hospitalized again. For years he refused aggressive care. Ultimately, his vision came to pass.

SOMETIMES A YOUNG PATIENT BEATS THE MEDIAN BY DECADES

Stephen Jay Gould was a highly regarded paleontologist, evolutionary biologist, historian of science, and popular science writer who died at age sixty from lung cancer. At age forty-one he was diagnosed with peritoneal mesothelioma, a rare cancer with a median life expectancy of eight months. Ultimately, rather than dying early, he survived nineteen years. His essay describing that experience, "The Median Isn't the Message," is considered a brilliant discussion of statistics, prognoses, and the difficulties of reconciling the individual patient and statistical averages in a humanistic discussion.[2]

Diagnosed with a rare cancer, he took a look at the survival curve of patients with abdominal mesothelioma and, rather than giving up because the left hand side of the median was short and the median survival itself was only eight months, he retained his innate optimism. He made note of the long tail of the survival to the right of the median (see figure 3). He embraced the concept that evolutionary biologists share "that variation itself is nature's only irreducible essence." Without specifically saying so, his essay implies that he "willed" himself into that long tail.

Inspired by the poetic genius of Dylan Thomas ("Do Not Go

3. The Median *Is* the Message

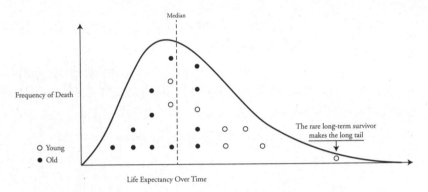

Figure 3. This represents a simple survival curve. If it were to represent the survival curve for abdominal mesothelioma in 1980, the median line would be situated at eight months. Note my addition: The solid dots, representing older patients, are clustered to the left of the median; and open circles, representing younger patients, are clustered to the right of the median. One younger patient is found to survive into the "long tail" of the curve.

Gentle into That Good Night") or William Ernest Henley's "Invictus" ("It matters not how strait the gate, how charged with punishment the scroll, I am the master of my fate, I am the captain of my soul"), one can see how the powerful human will to live is self-fulfilling. But when science is confused with poetic inspiration, we need a reality check. There are limits to the human will.

At no point in this book would I suggest that younger people decline potentially lifesaving or life-prolonging treatment. Gould, diagnosed at a young age, did not and should not have taken the median as the message without a fight. But to suggest that he willed his way to the long tail of the survival curve is poetic license rather than realistic thinking.

If my father had been diagnosed with mesothelioma at age ninety, I would have counseled him to refuse aggressive treatment and to enter hospice care. That is because for the elderly, the median is the message. The weak, old, and frail die before the median, and the young, initially strong, and subsequently lucky are more likely to survive into the long tail of the survival curve.

When dealing with disease and disability, will does play an important role. One can will oneself out of bed for another trial of chemo. One can will oneself to withstand multiple needle sticks or other painful procedures. One can will oneself to accept an attempt at heroic surgery. One can will oneself to tolerate the indignities of advanced debility and reliance on others for the basics of everyday living. But one cannot will where one will land on a statistical curve. One cannot will indefinite survival.

Fate is not subject to human will. Looking at a survival curve can inspire hope or despair. The hopeful will likely live longer than those who give up in despair. But we cannot will ourselves to land at a particular spot on that curve. That survival curve is created by the accumulation of thousands of clinical events in the treatment of any given illness. Most of these clinical events go well, but any one can turn disastrous. Rather than looking exclusively at the final shape of a survival curve, I think it is instructive to think of how that curve was developed, and a disk drop game (e.g., the Plinko board of *The Price is Right*) comes to my mind as an instructive visual image.

WHAT WE CAN LEARN FROM A DISK DROP GAME

In Plinko, a bonus round event in the long-running television show *The Price is Right* (now *The New Price is Right*), a contestant releases a chip from one of nine slots at the top of a board, hoping to drop the chip into one of nine slots at the bottom of the board that are associated with cash prizes. There are more than a hundred evenly distributed pegs between the top slots and the bottom slots.[3] Each chip strikes twelve pegs before landing at the bottom. At each peg the chip has a fifty-fifty chance of moving right or left. Ultimately each chip settles into a slot at the bottom of the board. In the world of TV disk drop, a single disk in the receiving slot represents a cash prize for the contestant. But if hundreds of disks were dropped through the same slot and allowed to accumulate at the bottom, a random distribution of disks would develop that was characteristic for each top slot.

In my concept of medical disk drop, the entrance slot represents the patient's diagnosis, the pegs represent medical interactions (surgeries, chemotherapy and radiation treatments, complications, infections, etc.), and the final slot represents the patient's life expectancy, which increases from left to right as seen in the survival curve of figure 3.

For each diagnosis a random distribution would follow as chip after chip is entered. Ultimately, each distribution would be reproducible for each diagnosis, but the path taken by every individual disk would be different. So here is the rub: each disk, or patient, has only one trip through the system, and where it ends up is a matter of fate and not will. It is possible that a patient can influence their diagnosis or entrance slot. Such an influence would usually be of the negative variety, for example, being a smoker increases the likelihood of entering the lung cancer slot.

Of course, medical therapies are designed to be effective, so each medical interaction has a risk–benefit ratio that is weighted toward the benefit side. But what would surprise most patients is how random medical outcomes can be. Complications of treatment occur even when everything is done routinely and done well. This randomness of complications validates the disk drop image.

Patients with seemingly easy-to-treat problems can crash and burn from the cancer or the treatment. Patients with "terminal illnesses" can live for a very long time. But these are rare outcomes. In general, the treatments work as intended. But because elderly patients begin treatments older and weaker than average, they tend to do less well than the median.

As an example of randomness, I remember, from many years ago, the curious juxtaposition of two colleagues in the medical staff lounge of my hospital. The older (but not old) man was a family practitioner and reformed smoker who had survived for years following surgery for pancreatic cancer at the Mayo Clinic. The younger colleague was a health-conscious gastroenterologist who never smoked and rarely drank. When the family practitioner left, I commented to my gastroenterology colleague that perhaps the Mayo Clinic had done well by the family practitioner. He responded, dismissively, suggesting that the diagnosis of pancreatic cancer was a mistake: "None of my patients have survived that long."[4] Ironically, and randomly, that second colleague developed pancreatic cancer himself and died ten months after the diagnosis and multiple aggressive treatments.

AGING PATIENTS OFTEN DO LESS WELL THAN THE MEDIAN

Statistically, elderly patients (here again, I mean chronically ill patients over the age of sixty-five or healthy patients over the average life expectancy for their demographic) will cluster below the median survival for a given disease for several reasons: many research trials are not designed for, or do not include, a large sample of aging patients; medical complexity increases with age; and Jefferson's vision of our skeletal structure breaking down like machinery applies to internal organs as well.[5]

When a research study is initiated, a group of patients is assembled. Members of the study group are usually enrolled over time, subjected to a treatment, and observed for results. The patients selected for a trial might be advanced in years, but they are not the sickest, most frail, most disease-ridden patients. The patients selected are chosen because they have less confounding illness and are expected to live long enough to measure the benefit of the treatment.

Therefore, when the median survival is determined for a research paper, it is not what one should expect for the frail and elderly patient discussing said treatment with a clinician.[6] In my mother's case, I knew from a search of the literature that stage IV lung cancer had a median survival of ten months. I also knew that at her age and with her weakness she was not likely to exceed the median survival. Indeed, despite limited treatment, she died in nine months.

MEDICAL COMPLEXITY

In this day and age there is considerable, and justifiable, focus on adverse medical outcomes. These are frequently lumped together and simply described as medical errors with little appreciation for the complexity of the intended treatment. Depending on the definition of a medical error (e.g., amputating the wrong leg) or an adverse event (e.g., a death following a heart transplant attempted on a complex, chronically ill, older patient), somewhere between 100,000 and 400,000 Americans die annually from the treatment they receive.[7] The larger number includes adverse outcomes that are considered unavoidable, but are still included as errors.

In the 1950s and 1960s there was an appreciation of, and an accepted diagnosis called, a "disease of medical progress." This was a reflection of the complexity of treatments as a result of the speed with which medical progress was occurring.[8] There is less focus on the concept of medical complexity now. However, medical complexity is the driving force behind the unpredictability of unavoidable errors.

You can intuitively grasp that the complexity of care increases with the number of diseases a patient has, the severity of their illnesses, the number of medications they take, the aggressiveness of the treatments they choose, and their age.

In the intensive care unit setting, where the most complicated patients are treated, unavoidable adverse incidents occur with regularity. Studies show that something goes seriously wrong every four or five days, more than half of those negative occurrences are unavoidable, 13 percent of them are fatal, and the majority of those who suffer fatal medical errors are elderly.[9]

AGING EXTENDS TO INTERNAL ORGANS

Most of us think of our muscles, tendons, and bones when Thomas Jefferson describes our machinery giving way with the loss of a pivot here or a pinion there (see epigraph, page 28). In our own world, we see muscles shrink and joints enlarge in our aging friends and relatives. We don't generally see or appreciate that the internal organs wear out in the same way, but they do.

We can observe the memory loss of dementia, but we don't envision the microscopic accumulation of debris in the connections between the nerve cells in the brain.

Other internal organs deteriorate without any external visible change, but the Jeffersonian principle is the same. The heart weakens as muscle fibers die and are replaced with scar tissue. The kidneys clog with debris as the nephrons (the microscopic filters) get blocked, one by one. The functional unit of the liver (the acinus) scars from inflammation caused by toxins (commonly alcohol and fat from excess dietary calories) and the lungs' tiny breathing sacks (alveoli) thicken or weaken from irritants (cigarette smoke and pollution). Blood vessel walls thicken with scar tissue following decades of pulsations causing stiffness and brittleness. The interior channels of our arteries narrow with fat and cholesterol deposits, changing flow patterns.

Previous medical therapies leave damage that comes back to haunt us. Radiation for breast cancer or lymphoma stiffens the arteries of neighboring tissue (including the heart tissue) and increases the chance of a heart attack years later. Chemotherapy targeted to cancers of the breast, blood, bladder, and bone can weaken the heart, kidneys, and liver. Those effects can be delayed and unpredictable.

The result of these invisible changes is the unpredictability of the old person's physiology that makes the effect of drugs, medications, manipulations, and surgeries unforeseeable.

A good friend and former patient suffered mightily when radiation he had for rectal cancer during his sixties caused a hole between his rectum and bladder following prostate cancer surgery in his seventies. Although appearing to be otherwise healthy and vigorous, he died during the surgery to repair that hole.

Most elderly people take multiple medications. Well before he stopped life-prolonging medications, at the peak of his participation in standard health care practices, my father was taking eight to ten types of pills and four ointments. This use of multiple medications has created the concept of polypharmacy.[10] In simple terms, polypharmacy means the more medications we use, the harder it is to predict the benefits or complications of their interactions.

But polypharmacy is a fact of life in our complicated medical world. If a seventy-year-old woman with diabetes, high blood pressure, osteoporosis, and asthma sees a physician, or a series of physicians, best practices dictate that she will be prescribed twelve medications. Instantly, she is placed in jeopardy of a medication complication.

Some patients think that taking more medications means better health care. Little do they know about the hidden dangers of medical complexity.

THE MEDIAN *IS* THE MESSAGE

Yes, we have had great advances in surgery and the treatment of leukemia and lymphoma. We have made intermediate progress with breast and prostate cancer. We have made less progress in the treatment of other solid cancers such as those of the lung, liver, pancreas, ovary, and brain. We are enjoying advances in the treatment of autoimmune diseases and heart disease. That is the good news. The bad news is that the progress we have made has not altered the inevitable. Everyone still dies of something.

The median is not the message that will be visited on you as an individual. Nor can a set of statistics be applied to each individual. But the median is the message that informs you of what is likely to happen. Use that understanding to your advantage.

If you think that you have lived "past the expiration date," then you are enjoying the first inkling of a reality check. Embrace it. Promoting aggressive medical treatment at that point increases the likelihood of prolonging a life of decreasing ability and diminishing returns. Transitioning to a more passive and accepting posture while actively refusing all but palliative care will give you as much control as possible.

For that reason, the median is the message, and acknowledging that is the alternative to magical thinking. Seeking less treatment is not "giving up." It is choosing a path that appears passive but is more natural and nurturing. Recognizing misguided hopefulness need not result in paralyzing hopelessness but can lead to peaceful purposefulness. If you recognize the median as the message, seize the day.

One of the attributes of a good death is to acknowledge that death and dying at an advanced age is appropriate.[11] Unburden your family. Share with them the peace of a decision to stop fighting. Avoid magical thinking and the inevitable failure of perpetually soldiering on. Replace misguided hope in the future with guided optimism and focus on the promise of the present.

I found much comfort in an acknowledgment of the appropriateness of his death when I stumbled on the obituary of a former professor, Farish Jenkins. I had written my undergraduate thesis with his guidance when he was a new paleontologist at Harvard. Physically and sartorially he looked like a nineteenth-century scholar sent from central casting. He died, at seventy-two, of pneumonia superimposed on recalcitrant multiple myeloma, a cancer of the blood and bone marrow. When I read his obituary, I was pleased to see that he had enjoyed an exceptionally good reputation with students and faculty alike. I was moved by a comment in his obituary that reflects how science, education, experience, or religion can help us put things in perspective. *The Economist* magazine reported that during his cancer treatment, he dismissed his visitors' worries, saying, "As a paleontologist, I am familiar with extinction."

My father engaged with his life. He did not engage with his illnesses. He calculated how to use his illness to his benefit, either to achieve a temporal goal such as surviving to meet his first great-granddaughter or to achieve a physical goal in the form of a quiet death at home.

Things to Remember/Things to Consider

- Create a vision of your death. Any vision, even one of dying from tobacco or alcohol abuse, becomes a point from which further understanding can develop.
- Internal organs age too, resulting in medical complexity and randomness of outcomes.
- You can will yourself to tolerate treatment; you cannot will the outcome of that treatment.
- Avoid magical thinking. The median *is* the message.
- Do not be afraid to discuss median survival for a serious diagnosis with your physician. Make them discuss it. If they dodge the subject, ask for a referral to a consultant who will discuss it.

Part Two

UNDERSTANDING
DISEASE

Chapter Five

How Different Diseases Lead to Common Causes of Death

Whether it is the anarchy of biochemistry or the direct result of its opposite—a carefully orchestrated genetic ride to death—we die of old age because we have been worn and torn and programmed to cave in.

—Sherwin B. Nuland, MD

Y OU DON'T HAVE to go to medical school to observe life and death. Medical school helps you understand the details of the process, but the broad brushstrokes are apparent to all thoughtful observers. Literature, scientific journals, and personal observations inform us of the arc of life as we ascend through youth, plateau in adulthood, and descend toward death.

This chapter will address the trajectory of disease as the arc of life makes that descent. I will describe the clinical course of illnesses by dividing them into acute and chronic categories. Within the category of chronic illness there are six diagnoses to which we attribute 90 percent of deaths among the elderly. I will sort through each of these processes and describe how each disease leads to death, finding that the six diseases share some common pathways. The goal is to help you to recognize the disease and trajectory with which you or your loved one is coping.

But first, let us start with my father. Technically, he died from the painless ravages of multiple small strokes, gradually losing his strength, mobility, dexterity, independence, and, finally, his will. Cerebrovascular disease (i.e., strokes—either multiple or solo) is one of those six leading causes of death. But to all outward appearances, he died of old age. This condition, old age (or more technically, senescence or frailty), is generally overlooked as a diagnosis. In reality, the progressive weakness of advanced age is created by our ability to postpone death by acute illness, and the result is that the body simply wears out.

Though he was eighty-six years old at the time, Dad did not die shortly after my mother did, as we, his children, had thought he might. He mourned, and then he persevered.

For three years after her death he engaged in his usual activities (French classes, water aerobics, personal training, the occasional social event, family milestones, reading, and correspondence) without apparent compromises. He regularly attended the movie theater broadcasts of the New York Metropolitan Opera's Saturday performances and made the rare theatrical reservation. He continued to drive himself as well as friends and neighbors to joint exercise classes.

More important, he continued to travel, both at home and abroad. Gradually, the travel started to become problematic. Planning trips began to include detailed studies of train platforms, steps, stairways, hotel room locations, and general issues of handicapped access. He was wearing diapers for long flights and using wheelchairs in airports.

His last airplane flights were five to six years after being widowed. He traveled to California in the care and company of my older sister and returned, several weeks later, accompanied by his host there, my middle sister. Although he considered traveling later that summer, plans went unmade or were canceled.

What went wrong? It turns out that he just got old.

OLD AGE AS A DIAGNOSIS

For the last five years of his life, my father had few major medical problems and no critical diagnoses. He took a blood pressure medicine, a cholesterol medication, various antidepressants of questionable benefit, and pain and anxiety pills, as needed. He was monitored for a chronic lymphoma, considered inactive except during his second to last summer. What he suffered from was fatigue, a progressive sapping of his strength that shrank his physical ability, and therefore his physical world.

This fatigue was analyzed from multiple different perspectives, but it defied further diagnosis. For several years we cycled him through a series of exams with his physicians. Each time the conclusions were the same. There was no convincing evidence of depression.[1] His internist said the fatigue was not metabolic, inflammatory, or hormonal based on multiple visits and the associated testing. His oncologist denied that the fatigue was the result of the lymphoma, which was deemed dormant. His cardiologist said that his heart was stronger than average for a man his age.

Finally, we recognized the pattern of serial and circular referrals for a problem that defied a diagnosis except that of old age. We all came to accept this as his slow downward trajectory, a gradual flight path to a bed-bound imprisonment.

About five years before he died, we started the process of hiring household help. At first, this included light housework and running errands with and without him. It progressed to include escorting him to the opera and theater. Ultimately we had to interweave formal outpatient nursing services. His household staff (college-age women and men seek-ing part-time work) took him to doctor's appointments and procedures. His nurses recorded and "translated" the interactions. Other nursing services were managing prescriptions and distributing medications to his pillboxes. Finally, he needed help with toileting and self-care.

In general, the fatigue of old age is hard to recognize and hard to acknowledge. Gradual appetite loss, decreased strength, and fatigue are more likely to be attributed to depression or, worse yet, a lack of will than to an actual physical illness known to the layperson only as old age. "I am too tired" sounds like a weakness of purpose rather than a hard-to-quantify symptom of disease.

As a practitioner, I can say that I saw it regularly. But as a gastro-enterologist, like other specialists, I did not have to focus on it. I could return most of those patients to their general medical physicians. "This patient's liver disease is not enough to explain their degree of fatigue," I would write in my consultation. The internist would then consult an endocrinologist for a thyroid-related explanation or a cardiologist for a heart failure explanation.

This might be because doctors don't want to accept a limit to their powers to diagnose and treat, and people don't want to accept weakness or fatigue as an acceptable or understandable part of old age. However, my father's persistent attempts to address it proved to us its existence.

A small part of the American medical establishment does recognize fatigue for what it is. Geriatricians define frailty as a clinical syndrome of three or more of the following symptoms: self-reported exhaustion (Dad's "fatigue"), unintentional weight loss, weakness (decreased grip strength, for example), slow walking speed, and low physical activity.[2]

To underscore the importance of this concept, this definition of frailty is independently predictive of falls, progressive disability, hospitalization, and death at two to four times the rate of the non-frail population.

About two years before his death, the demands of Dad's fatigue and weakness clashed with his desire to live independently. My sisters scheduled household help from eight a.m. to eight p.m. A year later, he fell several times in a single week while toileting himself during the night. It was clear at this point that my father was unable to live alone. After a family consultation, my older sister arranged twenty-four–seven coverage by incorporating the household assistants into a comprehensive outpatient nursing plan to include round-the-clock sitters or nursing assistants and regular nurse visits.

At this point Dad was using a transfer chair to get around outside of the apartment and a cane or a walker at home. He was getting some help in the shower. He was getting help tying his shoes. He needed help with straightening his clothes. We determined that he needed help with transferring from his bed to his chair. He was having rare but embarrassing "accidents." He was eating at the table without assistance.

Recognizing his poor performance status, Dad estimated it was time to stop visiting his remaining physicians. He called each one, thanked them for services rendered, and canceled future appointments. We discussed stopping his non-palliative medications. He chose not to at that moment. One month later he was admitted to hospice.

MORTAL TRAJECTORIES: PATTERNS OF DISEASE AND DYING

The arc of life and the trajectory of death have evolved dramatically just in the last century. During the peak of the Roman Empire the average life expectancy was thought to be less than thirty years old. At that time, infection, malnutrition, trauma, and occasionally other diseases combined to create an arc of life that was short and a trajectory of death best described as a ball rolling off a cliff at a comparatively young age. The same graph describes the trajectory of death from an

4. Loss of Performance Status

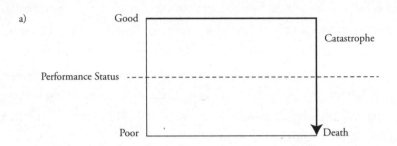

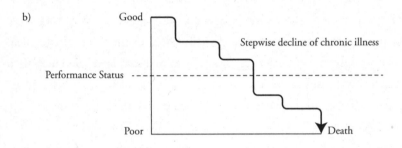

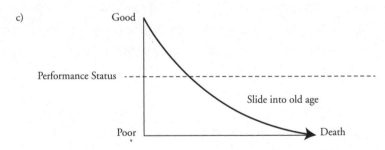

Figure 4. Three disease trajectories illustrating diminishing performance status for
a) catastrophe, b) chronic illness, and c) old age.

acute illness or event (an auto accident, for example) occurring at any age in our current era. (See figure 4a.)

People lived until they began to die, and when illness or trauma struck, death was fairly certain and quick.

In the Western world, life expectancy gradually increased with the advent of improved nutrition and the introduction of improved hygiene and sanitation. With the development of anesthesia and the surgical improvements of the late nineteenth century, further progress was made. But it was following the development of antibiotics, vaccines, diagnostic imaging, modern medical education, and the dissemination of medical information that life expectancy took off. Over the last several decades of the twentieth century, the average life expectancy in developed countries was increasing by two to three months per calendar year. But that rate has recently slowed, and there is no evidence to suggest that the current rate can be sustained.[3]

In the developed world, as fewer people are dying of acute illness, more people are dying of chronic illness. With that shift, the most common death trajectory curve changed from the drop described by a ball falling off of a cliff to the image of a ball stair-stepping down a plateaued hill. (See figure 4b.)

Patients could expect episodes of decline with successfully treated acute illnesses followed by periods of stable plateaus.

Finally, for a growing number of elderly patients, with chronic but stable disease, the slowly tapering decline of old age has become the final trajectory of death. This is how my father died. (See figure 4c.)

Let me briefly try to flesh out these patterns of decline, matching illnesses with the previous images and descriptions. Looking forward at the process is an exercise in recognizing a pattern that informs us what the future is likely to offer. Having an idea of what will come empowers us to think and invites planning.

PATTERNS OF ILLNESS: ACUTE ILLNESS

Tragedy occurs in a thousand different ways. Usually it is recognized in an acute illness (a bolt of lightning, an auto accident, or an overwhelming infection); sometimes it is seen in a slower process such as cancer at a young age or amyotrophic lateral sclerosis (ALS, commonly known as Lou Gehrig's disease). Occasionally it is perceived in the long, slow decline of the elderly.

Most acute illnesses rarely allow enough time to accommodate the kind of planning and decision making that I am promoting in this book. By definition, they come on suddenly and progress rapidly.

Examples of this type of acute illness include flesh-eating bacteria, meningitis, rampant pneumonia, trauma (from natural disasters, motor vehicle accidents, gun violence), stroke, or a heart attack at an unexpectedly young age. Most people probably know someone who survived such an acute ordeal. Fewer will have known someone who died at a young age of a disease commonly thought to be treatable. For those who do not, I offer Jim Henson, creator of Kermit the Frog and the Muppets, as an example.

Mr. Henson died at age fifty-three, in 1990, from complications of pneumonia. We generally think of pneumonia as treatable and curable. Antibiotics do cure most cases but not all. According to news reports, Mr. Henson took ill on a Saturday. He appeared to have the flu. He died less than a day later in the ICU of a New York City hospital. According to his doctor, the aggressive streptococcus that caused his pneumonia spread to the bloodstream (septicemia or sepsis) and subsequently caused liver and kidney failure.[4]

I can imagine the generic ICU scene that would have played out, usually over several days but in Mr. Henson's case in less than twenty-four hours. The eyes closed with tape and ointments; the breathing tube in the throat and the hiss of the ventilator, wheezing eighteen times per minute; the EKG monitor glowing green at the head of the bed; the portable hemodialysis unit at the foot of the bed, its circular pumps syphoning blood out and then back into the body; dozens of bags of fluid and medications hanging from IV poles, pumps blinking, feeding into a large vein in the neck or underneath the collar bone; the urinary catheter bag, hanging from the bed frame, slowly filling with unnaturally orange fluid; and the limbs tied to the bedframe to prevent accidental or reflexive removal of any of the intruding tubes are images common to this ICU scenario.

For a patient at age fifty-three, this acute process plays out of necessity. Treatment after treatment is piled on until recovery begins or death supervenes. This aggressive treatment is appropriate. There is no time or desire to think about slowing down. In the young, formerly healthy, patient, acute disease demands acute treatment. There is no pattern to consider. There is no reason to pause. Yet this is not necessarily the case when acute illness is superimposed on the chronic illness of an elderly patient.

The Centers for Disease Control and Prevention (CDC) recognizes four acute diagnoses that account for the deaths of about 10 percent of people over the age of sixty-five. These are unintentional injury (think falls), influenza and pneumonia (think Jim Henson at an older age), nephritis (think kidney failure), and septicemia (think overwhelming infection without an apparent source).

Eighty percent of elderly people suffer a fall, with or without injury, sometime, some way. According to the CDC, more than 3 percent of elderly people die as a direct result of traumatic injury, most of which is precipitated by these falls. Those who do not die, but are injured, suffer variable degrees of long-term damage.

In chapter 2, I described an elderly woman with late-onset ulcerative colitis who died of pneumonia in the ICU after attempts to treat her colon with an immune suppressant. Demographically, she would be clumped in the influenza and pneumonia group.

Death by acute kidney failure (nephritis) can usually be prevented by hemodialysis. But at an advanced age, when long-term dialysis is inappropriate, 3 percent of older Americans die as a result.

And septicemia, as a stand-alone diagnosis, causes death among 2 percent of the elderly population when they arrive at the hospital in a state of shock, an unexpected infection of the blood is found, and no other diagnosis or source for the infection can be determined to explain the process.

To a person, these elderly patients have died of an acute illness. Most of them will have died hospitalized deaths, some in the intensive care unit, while their collapse is being diagnosed and treated. But with some planning and enough foresight, the location of those deaths might have been modified to something more comfortable and less isolated. I will say more on that later in this chapter, as well as in chapters 6 and 8.

Now, let us move on to the most common chronic diagnoses that cause death in the elderly.

PATTERNS OF DISEASE: CHRONIC ILLNESSES, OR HOW WE DIE, AN UPDATED PERSPECTIVE

Six chronic diseases (congestive heart failure, cancer, chronic obstructive pulmonary disease, stroke, dementia, and diabetes) are responsible for, or credited with, causing 90 percent of the deaths among Americans over the age of sixty-five. Yes, no matter how healthy you feel at age sixty-five, demographically speaking, the Centers for Disease Control's Division of Vital Statistics groups you with the octogenarians and above.[5] A brief description of each illness follows.

Congestive Heart Failure (Responsible for about 34 Percent of Deaths over Sixty-Five)

Congestive heart failure (CHF) is the most common cause of death in the elderly. Nearly 500,000 people over the age of sixty-five die of CHF each year. It is a chronic illness with a pattern of recurrent hospitalizations ending with a self-perpetuating downward spiral. It is the result of ineffective pumping because of some combination of muscle weakness and heart valve malfunction. Tight valves cause the strain of back-pressure. Loose valves lead to increased backflow, chamber enlargement, and the increased work. Muscle weakness can be the direct result of viruses, toxic medications, or autoimmune processes. However, the cumulative effects of large and small heart attacks explain the majority of cases.

CHF usually starts indirectly, with atherosclerosis (hardening of the arteries from high cholesterol and chronic inflammation). Atherosclerotic cardiovascular change is almost universal in those who eat the average American diet. It simply depends on how hard we look for the pathological changes. When advanced changes are present, the disease begins the process of muscle damage with cell fallout or muscle death caused by the oxygen deprivation of narrowed blood vessels. Tiny blood vessel blockage leads to microscopic areas of cell death. Larger vessel blockage leads to larger areas of cell death known as a myocardial infarction (heart attack). All cell death leads to replacement by fibrosis (scar tissue) and progressive weakness of the muscle wall.

Heart valves can be replaced, if one is strong enough to tolerate the surgery and the attendant problems of artificial valves. Blockages of large arteries can be opened with balloons or stents. But, again, damage cannot reliably be reversed and, whereas rehabilitation can improve existing heart muscle, generation of new muscle does not occur.

At some point, the accumulation of muscle loss leads to ineffective pumping. This is when heart failure appears. Diminished outflow from the heart changes the flow dynamics recorded by the kidneys. Perceiving less flow, the kidneys retain water. Increased backflow from the heart aggravates this. Fluid accumulates in the lungs, abdomen, and legs. Fluid in the lungs causes shortness of breath. Fluid in the legs causes skin breakdown. Fluid in the abdomen is generally cosmetic but in excess it decreases breathing, increases work, and promotes inactivity.

At first this process can be postponed with diuretics (water pills) and heart medications. Frequently, hospitalization is required to improve breathing, rid the body of excess fluid, and readjust the heart pills. The chance of pneumonia is increased by the presence of water-logged lungs. Pneumonia is frequently hard to distinguish from simple CHF and then presumptive use of antibiotics becomes part of the treatment.

Objective measurements of heart size, wall motion, and ejection fraction (the percent of blood that is ejected with each heartbeat) are safely, easily, and accurately obtained with ultrasound-like equipment that is available in every hospital and cardiologist's office. Not an electrocardiogram (EKG), which records the heart's electrical impulses, the echocardiogram uses sound waves to create two and three-dimensional images of the valves, chambers, and walls. Measurements of these structures can be compared over time and inferences can be drawn about the progress of the disease. Patients can be advised when the situation is becoming critical either by monitoring this objective data or observing the pattern of increasingly frequent hospitalizations.

Death by CHF is commonly the result of respiratory failure caused by fluid that is retained in the lungs or concurrent pneumonia. This may be accompanied by simultaneous kidney or liver failure. It is less commonly caused by a disturbance in the heart's rhythm, because of the increased use of implantable pacemakers and defibrillators. Death is usually predicted by a cycle of increased symptoms, deterioration, hospitalization, medication adjustment, stabilization, and then increased symptoms again. When the cyclical pattern of doctor visit, progressive dysfunction (as measured by serial echocardiograms), hospitalization, medication change, and overall deterioration is recognized, some patients might choose to refuse hospitalization and seek palliative care. For more on palliative care, see chapter 11.

Cancer (Responsible for about 28 Percent of Deaths over Sixty-Five)

Cancer is an umbrella term that encompasses hundreds of diseases and diagnoses characterized by uncontrolled cell growth. Cancer is the second most common cause of death among the aging and elderly, killing just over 400,000 older people annually. Death from various cancers can be so varied as to defy simplified characterization. Some people hemorrhage to death. Some people choke to death. The spread of cancer to the brain (metastases) can lead to intractable seizures and cause death by increased intracranial pressure (brain swelling). Cancers within the abdomen and pelvis will obstruct the bowel. Malnutrition contributes to many cancer deaths, although thankfully the concurrent loss of appetite spares the patient from the symptoms of starvation.

Because of poor nutrition, weakened immune systems, resistant organisms, and complications of treatment, most patients will finally die of (or with) infections such as pneumonia, urinary tract infections, and abscesses, among others. But, unlike the other chronic illnesses, cancer deaths are frequently associated with significant pain problems as the tumor, or its metastases, infiltrate bones, compress adjacent organs, inflame nerves, or block the bowels.

Another cruel truth about cancer is that the treatment is frequently difficult to bear and fraught with complications. Surgery hurts. Radiation therapy and chemotherapy inflame tissues, induce fatigue, and nauseate patients.

Cancers should be fought aggressively until such time as they should be fought no further. That point is defined by the confluence of multiple factors. Perhaps it is the recognition that successive treatment options are progressively ineffective and that the decline is irreversible. For, when the pain is debilitating, when scans and X-rays show progression of the disease despite aggressive therapies, when multiple systems become involved, and when the will to struggle on is weakened by the observable reality, then the time to fight is past and the time to focus on symptom control through palliation has arrived. I will leave further discussion of this chronic illness to the chapter dealing with how to recognize a terminal illness (chapter 8)

Chronic Obstructive Pulmonary Disease (Responsible for about 9 Percent of Deaths over Sixty-Five)

Chronic obstructive pulmonary disease (COPD) is the catchall phrase for chronic lung disorders, the most common of which are emphysema (loss of alveoli—the small breathing sacs) and bronchitis (inflamed airways). COPD kills about one quarter the number of patients who die of CHF.

The most common cause of COPD is smoking tobacco products. However, every subset of lung disease can occur independent of tobacco use. Inhalation of other toxins can mimic tobacco damage. Emphysema can be genetic. Adult onset asthma can lead to chronic bronchitis. Bronchitis can lead to spastic narrowing of the airways or destructive widening of the airways (bronchiectasis). Interstitial lung disease, a thickening of all lung tissue of unknown cause, combines elements of both emphysema and bronchitis. All of these pathological processes lead to poor drainage of mucus and irritants with recurrent infections and progressive damage.

Although there are some diagnosis-specific treatments for the various forms of COPD, there is no specific cure or antidote. Treatments can slow progression and improve symptoms, but none repair damage.

Unlike that which occurs in some organs, lung regeneration is non-existent. One hallmark of this chronic disease is recurrent episodes of pneumonia or bronchitis. Antibiotics are initially successful to treat these infections and may remain so for years. Another hallmark is the hard work and energy that COPD patients must expend to continue breathing. This results in significant weight loss from excess caloric expenditure.

Eventually, however, problems arise. Side effects occur, secondary infections such as *Clostridia difficile* colitis develop, resistant respiratory organisms arise, and progressive weakness from inactivity and bed rest becomes evident.

Lung function is easily and effectively measured. This means the deterioration of COPD can be accurately monitored. Most important, doctors should advise, and patients should understand, that the recurrent infections and progressive damage become a self-fulfilling process. When this downward spiral is recognized, and certain milestones of lung dysfunction are reached, the terminal nature of the disease must be acknowledged.

Recognizing a pattern of decreasing pulmonary function, increasing supplemental oxygen requirements, and diminishing performance status might inform future clinical decisions.

Absent a superimposed acute illness or complication, death from COPD will be respiratory in nature. Patients will get a pneumonia that resists treatment or will simply fade away from lack of oxygen. In either event the symptoms can be palliated with morphine, and the actual death will be comparatively comfortable, whether the patient waits until the very end or hastens the process by declining antibiotics or demanding more opiates.

An unfortunate scenario that occurs frequently enough with end-stage COPD patients is the juxtaposition of an acute surgical emergency on the chronic respiratory decline. If a COPD patient has a bowel obstruction, appendicitis, or a gallbladder attack, for example, the decision to operate can be a difficult one. Most abdominal surgery requires an endotracheal tube to administer general anesthesia. Because COPD patients, exhausted by the work of breathing, rapidly become reliant on mechanical ventilation, even an hour on the breathing machine in the operating room can commit the patient to days, or weeks, on the ventilator in the post-op ICU without guarantee of recovery. This prolonged intubation and bed rest do guarantee further problems, deterioration, and debility. Although most bowel obstructions are miserable, declining surgery at this point might result in less suffering in the long run.

Added together, the next three major chronic illnesses (stroke, dementia, and diabetes) cause only about one quarter of the deaths caused by the first three chronic illnesses, although they may contribute mightily to the degree of disability of any decline.

Cerebrovascular Disease—AKA Stroke (Responsible for about 8 Percent of Deaths over Sixty-Five)

To describe cerebrovascular disease as one of the chronic illnesses that results in death requires some explanation. Most laypeople know at least one person with a one-off stroke. A surprise occurrence resulting in a palsied arm, leg, or face and some degree of speech difficulty, this one-time episode is not usually fatal and is commonly followed by some degree of recovery. This type of stroke might be the result of a blood clot originating in the heart, an abnormal blood vessel in the brain, or a unique area of cholesterol plaque. It might not be the result of advanced, systemic disease.

While stroke is the fourth most common cause of death among elderly Americans, it is the second most common cause of death and the third most common cause of disability worldwide. There are slightly fewer than 800,000 strokes per year in the United States, of which 600,000 are primary and 200,000 are recurrent. These numbers do not include the micro-strokes or transient ischemic attacks (TIAs) that go unnoticed or resolve quickly and that usually indicate underlying atherosclerosis (hardening of the arteries) with the likelihood of future clinical events.

Eighty percent of strokes are caused by decreased blood flow. Most commonly this is the result of atherosclerosis. Twenty percent of strokes result from bleeding within the head, either in the brain tissue or around it.

If a large stroke does not cause immediate death, the disability that occurs may indirectly lead to death or contribute to deterioration. Complications of bed rest and swallowing disorders with choking are two obvious results.

Less well known among the lay public is the process of multiple strokes that progress below the level of the clinically obvious. Tiny strokes (micro-infarcts) that occur below the cortex (the surface of the brain) are called lacunar strokes. They may not cause an immediately definable event but have a cumulative effect leading to neuromuscular deterioration and multi-infarct dementia.

My father's last few months were punctuated with small strokes. His caregivers occasionally reported a sudden weakness in an arm or leg. On my last visit I noticed that he would eat meals using only his right hand (he was right-hand dominant) despite dropping his food and fork with regularity. If reminded to use his left hand he would do so tentatively. This type of spatial neglect (hemi-agnosia) was almost certainly the result of a tiny stroke.

Therefore, cerebrovascular disease can occur suddenly or creep up slowly. If not immediately fatal, it leads to chronic changes and weakness with the self-perpetuating deterioration of the wheelchair-bound or bed-bound elderly. The prognosis of patients with cerebrovascular disease is harder to determine than with CHF or COPD. All but massive strokes allow the potential for recovery, but there is no way to predict when recovery from a single stroke will end. The long-term prognosis in cerebrovascular disease is difficult to grasp because the decline is functional and partly subjective, unlike the objective changes of the heart's ejection fraction or the lungs' volume. In my experience, once multiple tiny strokes are recognized, they tend to recur at an accelerated pace. Again, recurrent hospitalizations for aspiration pneumonia, blood clots, or catheter-induced urinary infections define the glide path to death. Analyses of frailty and performance status by a geriatrician might offer other insights for patients and proxies to discuss. When recurrent complications and a cycle of deterioration are recognized, seeking palliative care is appropriate.

Dementia (Responsible for about 6 Percent of Deaths over Sixty-Five)

Dementia is a very common chronic illness. It is age related. The longer one lives, the more likely he or she will suffer some degree of dementia. Nearly half of people over age eighty-five have some degree of dementia in addition to some other chronic illness. However, it is much less commonly the primary chronic illness that is listed as the cause of death on the death certificate.

Dementia is another catchall phrase for a variety of conditions that lead to cognitive impairment, but in our daily lexicon "dementia" more frequently means Alzheimer's disease. Unless otherwise speci-fied, that is how I will use it here. It is uniformly fatal, and its course can be plotted in the same way the five-year survival of every cancer is monitored for prognostic and research purposes.

However, dementia, in particular Alzheimer's, merits additional consideration. Appendix II, a section of specialized information in the back matter, will address the extra planning that dementia requires. Here I will address how dementia kills.

Almost everyone has a personal connection to someone suffering from dementia. This familiarity, however, is deceptively incomplete, because patients with advanced dementia tend to be socially isolated or institutionalized. Assailed with the promotion of Alzheimer's care units, advertisements promising new treatments, and politicians' guarantees of funding successful research programs, people might think that real progress is being made in the treatment and prevention of the illness. If you define "real progress" as minimal and incremental, then you are correct.

Alzheimer's disease is a comparatively virulent form of dementia that is clinically divided into early-onset (strong genetic component) versus late-onset (multifactorial origin). Late-onset Alzheimer's cases are growing as the aging population grows.

Medical professionals regularly divide Alzheimer's into stages. Early, middle, and late stages are commonly used to categorize the illness for purposes of determining competence, level of care requirements, and prognosis.

Dementia first steals the memory of the immediate past, then the present, then the distant past, then the patient's personality, and finally the soul. Following the mental decline is a late physical decline resulting in bedridden, noncommunicative vessels of former persons who do not understand the activities of daily living, not to mention the medical tests, that caregivers and medical personnel force on them.

Early stage patients are described as forgetful. They are competent and can be left alone and in a self-care situation. Their prognosis is measured in years. Middle-stage patients segue from competent to incompetent. They transition from self-care to requiring companions to protect them from themselves. They are characterized by getting lost and being dangerously forgetful. They forget where they are in time and place. Their prognosis is also measured in years. Late stage patients are incompetent. They do not recognize close family members. They might not know who they are. Eventually they suffer degenerative changes of the peripheral nerves, leading to weakness and dysfunction of the extremities, throat, and respiratory muscles. These changes bear some similarities to other neurodegenerative diseases such as ALS or advanced Parkinson's disease. The prognosis for late stage dementia is measured in many months to several years.

Therefore, death from Alzheimer's can result from trauma incurred from wandering abroad or falling down familiar stairs; poison consumed; mistaken dosages of medicine; or myriad other insults visited upon those who cannot think clearly, remember accurately, or protect themselves. Most commonly, those patients who live into the late stages of the disease die of pneumonia or other infections after multiple episodes of choking and aspiration.

Although their deaths usually follow the predictable physical decline of other degenerative diseases of the nervous system, the late stage demented patient is incompetent and cannot speak for him or herself when the need is the greatest. To make decisions that might lead to palliation and avoid painful medical interventions that the demented patient does not understand, agents need to have discussed and understood that patient's wishes in advance of their incompetence.

Diabetes Mellitus (Responsible for about 4 Percent of Deaths over Sixty-Five)

Diabetes mellitus (DM) comes in two forms. Type 1 diabetes (commonly known as "insulin-dependent" and formerly known as "juvenile diabetes") is a common, chronic illness that does exist in old age, but it is not the prominent form of diabetes in the elderly. The most common form of diabetes in the elderly is Type 2 diabetes. Obesity, insulin resistance, and a worn-out pancreas cause this type. Sometimes insulin is required to manage the high blood sugar levels, but most patients are managed with oral medication and various non-insulin injectables.

Type 2 diabetes is a systemic disease that causes the deterioration of multiple organs and systems. In isolation, it is less likely to be the sole cause of death, but it contributes to multiple other fatal pathways.

The high blood sugar levels of type 2 diabetes contribute to more virulent infections. They also contribute to small blood vessel changes of atherosclerosis (hardening of the arteries). These changes result in mini-strokes and mini–heart attacks. Atherosclerosis in the kidneys leads to decreased renal function and eventually to renal failure. This complicates fluid retention and electrolyte balance.

Atherosclerosis and high blood sugars cause peripheral nerve damage leading to insensitivity of the feet and ankles. This in turn leads to increased falls. Microvascular damage in the extremities leads to poor circulation, skin breakdown, infection, and gangrene.

The associated obesity causes resistance to blood flow and complications of high blood pressure. Fat deposits in the liver lead to inflammation, fibrosis (mild scarring), and cirrhosis (advanced scarring).

In summary, type 2 diabetes causes accelerated damage to all the organs subject to the ravages of atherosclerosis (brain, heart, kidneys, and blood vessels) as well as liver dysfunction and peripheral nerve damage. Although rarely the direct and sole cause of death, type 2 diabetes is a secondary contributor to a large percentage of deaths in the aged. When a physician is called to the coronary care unit to pronounce a patient dead from a heart attack, if there is a history of stroke, dialysis, amputation, or non–alcohol induced cirrhosis then you can be sure that "complications of diabetes" will appear on the death certificate.

Therefore, death from diabetes can be the result of accelerated heart failure, kidney failure, or infection. Or death can be the result of a diabetic coma from one of two causes: a dramatically reduced blood sugar (too much insulin) or a dramatically elevated blood sugar with dehydration and accumulated toxins (ketoacidosis) because of inadequate insulin. Like other comatose states, diabetic coma is a comparatively comfortable way to die.

OLD AGE AS A CHRONIC DISEASE

Having just reviewed some observations about the six major categories of chronic illness and the trajectories of their progression, I would like to volunteer "old age" as a common diagnosis that should be considered more than a condition and included in every calculation related to a patient's treatment and prognosis.

Sherwin Nuland, in his classic, award-winning book *How We Die* [6] described death as a process and forcefully wrote that his grandmother died of old age over an eighteen-year period, not just of the "cerebrovascular accident" listed on her death certificate. He wrote, "Though their doctors dutifully record such distinct entities as stroke, or cardiac failure, or pneumonia, these aged folk have in fact died because something in them has worn out."

I assert that old age is both a process and a disease state. It steals the life of elderly people as predictably as any of the six chronic diseases. Perhaps it does so because every elderly person without a predominant illness is likely to have a little bit of several of the chronic illnesses.

My father was an excellent case in point. At the time that I began writing this book he was ninety-three years old and living a bed-to-chair existence in his apartment with round-the-clock staff. Although he had a history of high blood pressure and had undergone a cardiac catheterization (almost thirty years before), he had never suffered a heart attack, nor was he diagnosed with CHF. Yet his aortic aneurysm was proof that he had hardening of the arteries. He had not smoked since his service in the Second World War, but we might have found decreased lung function if we had chosen to test for it. He was not clinically demented. He had cancer in the form of a chronic lymphoma that was causing no obvious problems. He had dry skin, a peripheral neuropathy, exertional shortness of breath, minimal short-term memory loss, and debilitating fatigue. No doctor was able to attribute his functional limitations or his fatigue to any one of the six chronic illnesses. Yet he had elements of five of the six chronic illnesses (there is no evidence of diabetes and he had never been overweight), and all that everyone could agree on was that he was really old. Because his decline was inexplicably and, at times, agonizingly slow, it was easy to overlook the incremental changes and the subtle contributions of each of his conditions.

Geriatricians measure old age with a variety of yardsticks. Frailty is measured in physical parameters such as weight loss, grip strength, and nutritional status. Other measures relate to performance status.

The Karnofsky Performance Status (KPS) is one such example of a measure that assesses overall performance, particularly with respect to cancer treatments and survivability.[7] A low KPS should prompt questions about the appropriateness of aggressive therapy.

In addition to overall performance status, there are a host of activities of daily living assessments to choose from.[8] These are tools that geriatricians and clinical social workers use to quantify the ability to bathe, dress, toilet, transfer from bed to chair, maintain continence, and eat. You can imagine that as frailty and performance are quantified, scores can be established, a pattern can be recognized, and a prognosis can be estimated.

My sisters and I did not need to graph our father's decline to recognize the appropriate time for hospice care, but others might benefit by doing so.

CASE STUDIES

I would like to describe two examples of former patients whose deaths or diseases exemplify the downward spiral of chronic disease and old age.

JOHN: CONGESTIVE HEART FAILURE

One such scenario unfolded like this. John, a seventy-eight-year-old retired executive, had mild congestive heart failure. A former smoker, heavy social drinker, and type 2 diabetic, John caught the flu in January, eighteen months before I left my practice. He was initially bedridden by the muscle aches and weakness of the viral infection; progressive coughing and the production of green phlegm heralded the arrival of a bacterial pneumonia. He was hospitalized in the ICU, where he responded well to his IV fluid and antibiotic treatment. However, mild liver dysfunction and early kidney disease from diabetes caused fluid retention in the chest and abdomen. This compromised his breathing and mobility. After a few days in the ICU and a week on the medical floor, he was unable to stand and walk alone. A few weeks in a nursing home allowed for some degree of rehabilitation, and he returned home on a host of new medicines to keep the fluid off and to regulate his electrolytes and heart rhythm. In March, because of low potassium and magnesium, he developed atrial fibrillation. This was unrecognized for some time, and the rapid heart rate compromised the oxygenation of his heart muscle, resulting in a small heart attack and worsened heart failure.

Over the next eight months John required a series of emergency room visits and more than one hospitalization, sometimes for fluid overload from heart failure, sometimes for cardiac rhythm disturbances, sometimes for dehydration from medications or diarrhea. Occasionally he required nursing home placement to rehabilitate his weak heart and leg muscles. With each hospitalization he lost some ground in terms of strength and independence. By the next January he was essentially house-bound and limited to a single-floor existence. His trips to the hospital had the feeling of a revolving door. His time in the nursing home led him to believe that long-term residence there was not of interest to him.

John's downhill slide ended with the heart failure diagnosis. In retrospect there were multiple chronic illnesses that contributed to the process, including heart disease, lung disease, diabetes, liver disease, and kidney disease. John and his wife, both longtime patients, recognized the pattern of deterioration in the winter of my last year in practice. They realized that recurrent shortness of breath, repeat courses of antibiotics for pneumonia, multiple medication adjustments for fluid accumulation, and readmissions to hospitals and nursing homes predicted future problems. He entered hospice that spring and died quietly thereafter, declining antibiotics for pneumonia but taking morphine and oxygen for respiratory failure.

PATRICK: CANCER AND CHRONIC LUNG DISEASE

Another example that comes to mind is that of Patrick, a surprisingly laconic Brooklyn-born Irishman. I assume he was born into a working-class background based on his education and early career. When I met him he was a successful lobbyist in DC and a charming gentleman. His gastrointestinal issues were quite mundane and not memorable, but his slide into chronic illness was, and it began with interstitial lung disease. This is a disease caused by a disordered immune system that progressively thickens the lung tissue and suffocates the patient. The process can be slowed, but a cure, or reversal, depends on receiving a lung (or a heart-lung) transplant. His career came to a halt as his disease progressed. Then advancing age and a second diagnosis (acute leukemia) destroyed his chance at a possible transplant. He died at age seventy-five of his combined illnesses.

I remember his gradual decline, his visits to my office in a wheelchair, attached to his supplemental oxygen. His phlegmatic demeanor never changed. His wife or daughter was always in attendance. Yet his hair loss, his abdominal complaints, his pallor (anemia), his weight loss, and his weakness spoke volumes to me about the struggles he was experiencing with his continued chemotherapy. He ultimately died while still pursuing a cure for his leukemia long after that goal was possible. Whether he recognized the pattern of his decline and yet chose to fight it or whether he did not see the inevitable is unclear to me. I think he chose to fight because that was who he was. The result was prolonged suffering and a hospitalized death. I was not his primary care physician and could only advise tangentially.

His wife, Marilyn, died a few years later at home in hospice care. She remembered Patrick's treatment and recognized the pattern of his decline—chemotherapy, complications, side effects, and debility—in the care of her own uterine cancer. She chose early hospice admission. This was a common sequence of events. The first spouse dies after too much painful, costly, and futile care and the trailing spouse chooses to enter hospice care at the earliest appropriate time.

RECOGNIZING PATTERNS

In the previous sections I have painted a picture of how acute illnesses differ from chronic illnesses and how chronic illnesses frequently follow predictable patterns.

I have introduced you to the relatively few diseases that are responsible for 90 percent of the deaths in Americans over the age of sixty-five. An understanding of these diseases is manageable. An appreciation of how they progress is possible. Recognizing a pattern in their clinical course is empowering. When these diseases follow recognizable patterns, and if you choose to avoid medicalization, death arrives in one of a few, more predictable, ways.

As exemplified by the preceding stories, these six chronic illnesses are not mutually exclusive. Two or more of these chronic illnesses can combine to create minor variations in how the disease progresses, but they still tend to offer a recognizable pattern of symptom, treatment, complication, decline, plateau; symptom, treatment, complication, decline, plateau; and so on until the process leads to frailty.

What we do when we recognize that pattern dictates whether we choose a medicalized death or a more peaceful death.

Of course, we grieve when we lose something dear, including some aspect of our health. We despair when we recognize that each treatment cycle results in less benefit and more deterioration. But we are empowered when we can see that when treatment is increasingly ineffective, then treatment is no longer the only option and comfort care might be a better choice. When we make that choice we take control away from the doctors and return it to ourselves.

These decisions should be based on knowledge about the downhill course of the disease, not on the false hope of a long-term reprieve. They should be made with the understanding that some patients who choose comfort care (palliative care) will live longer than those who choose aggressive treatments and, more important, all patients who choose palliative care will be more comfortable.

CHOOSING COMFORT OVER CYCLICAL TREATMENT: HAVING A VISION

In arguing against the repair of his aortic aneurysm, my father asked me, "Why would I fix something that will carry me away the way I want to go?" He had a vision of one kind of death, and he was trying to articulate a plan.

To the degree that people consider their death at all, most people would prefer a quick and painless death. Their vision is to die in their sleep. Certainly my father preferred the idea of a pain-free passage. But he was also practical, and he did not want to reflexively close the door on another quick option such as an aneurysm failure.

To die in your sleep, in fact to die at all in the presence of advanced chronic disease, you have to assume that something acute occurs. This could be a ruptured aneurysm (or some other potential surgical emergency), a giant stroke, a heart attack, or a blood clot to the lungs. As visions go, these events are quick, but they are unpredictable. Infections, however, are common enough among the old and infirm to offer some degree of reproducibility and predictability. Yet few people include them in their vision because we perceive of infections as eminently treatable. And, like so many other treatment decisions, when something is treatable we feel obligated to try.

Pneumonia and bladder infections are familiar to almost everyone. But there are many other kinds of infections that most people do not think about. Nearly every kind of infection that might cause pain can also occur in a painless form. As a gastroenterologist I saw more cases of painless bile duct infections than painful ones. I also saw many cases of painless colon infections (diverticulitis) despite its reputation as a painful condition. The real point to take home is that painless infections, untreated, will lead to an overwhelming infection. And an overwhelming infection, palliated, is a comparatively quick and comfortable way to die.

Let's look more closely at deathbed scenarios in the next chapter.

Things to Remember/Things to Consider

- Disease can be characterized; the course of disease can be observed; an understanding can be developed.
- Consider "old age" to be a diagnosis.

- Discuss the course of your particular chronic illness with your physician.
- Recognize the pattern of recurrent symptoms, treatment, deterioration, and stabilization.
- If you recognize a cycle of unproductive treatment and progressive decline, consider refusing treatment that prolongs a painful dying process.

Chapter Six

Deathbed Scenarios: How Does the End Finally Arrive?

First I will define what I conceive medicine to be. In general terms, it is to do away with the suffering of the sick, to lessen the violence of their disease, and to refuse to treat those who are overmastered by their diseases, realizing that in such cases medicine is powerless.

— Hippocrates, *The Art,* Corpus Hippocraticum

HOW DOES THE end finally arrive? That depends on when "finally" is defined to begin or how far back we move away from the last breath and the final heartbeat. But let's face it: some medical professionals want us to believe that the dying process is so complicated that we must leave it in their hands. In the last chapter I focused on the trajectories of the six common chronic diseases responsible for the deaths of 90 percent of elderly patients. The goal was to achieve an understanding of the course of those illnesses and then to recognize patterns that predicted the failure of future treatments. In deference to our trusted medical professionals, let us acknowledge that the treatment of those illnesses is complicated, but let us also acknowledge that the outcome, if not perfectly straightforward, is inevitable. In this chapter I will examine death certificates to further simplify the dying process and to highlight points for decision making. Ultimately we want to visualize a series of events that moves toward a more comfortable death.

The fact that the CDC's Department of Vital Statistics organizes 90 percent of elder deaths into six categories of chronic illness is useful to our simplification process. But, for the moment, let us stop looking at how a disease progresses and look at the very end of a life instead, trying to dissect the final phase of the disease process and establish some commonalities that occur on every deathbed.

DEATH CERTIFICATES AND WHAT THEY ILLUMINATE

Death certificates are a thumbnail sketch of a patient's disease and the dying process. When properly filled out, these documents outline the sequence and the time line of the clinical events that result in death. Therefore, examining death certificates offers a different perspective for understanding this final phase.

What is common to every death, but excluded from use on a death certificate, is that the heart stops beating and the lungs stop ventilating, in no particular order, but in rapid succession. Cardiorespiratory arrest is the universal medical event that ultimately defines the physical state of death, so cardiac arrest, respiratory arrest, and cardiorespiratory arrest are terms that do not inform the authorities. They are generally excluded from death certificates. Instead, the death certificate should reflect the sequence of diseases that describes the terminal arc and brings us to the point of cardiorespiratory arrest. Developing a sense of that disease sequence maximizes the chances of approaching death with less pain and without prolongation.

Also common to, but unmentioned in, every death certificate is a period of unconsciousness before the last breath or the last heartbeat. This unconsciousness may last a few moments following the collapse of a heart attack, a few days following the coma of dehydration or the sleepiness of overwhelming infection, or months to years following brain damage. Medical personnel understand that a coma itself is painless. Therefore, aiming to create the circumstances for a deep coma sets the stage for a comparatively good, comparatively quiet death.

MY FATHER'S DEATH CERTIFICATE

I have filled out many death certificates. I never lost the sense of responsibility to be associated with the process. Actuaries, coders, statisticians, researchers, and family members will forever use what a doctor writes on the certificate to process, record, analyze, understand, and comfort, respectively. It is a solemn moment sandwiched between the pronouncement of the body and its transfer to the morgue or the funeral home. It is a moment that codifies the covenant between the doctor's care and demographic eternity.

Every death certificate contains a huge amount of information. The patient's name, address, age, date of birth, ethnicity, occupation, aliases, Social Security number, education, marital status, and armed forces service are recorded for statistical follow-up. What challenges the medical professional finishing the form and adding the dramatic context is the cause of death. This is because every death certificate requests three or four diagnoses, placed in series and along a time line, to establish a cause of death. The goal is to create a chain of events consisting of the diseases or complications that occurred in sequence to result in death.

The medical section of a generic death certificate would have this format:

The conditions listed are the diseases, injuries, or complications that caused death. Conditions leading to the immediate cause are listed sequentially and the underlying cause is listed last.

Cause of death—do not enter terminal events such as cardiac or respiratory arrest.

    a. Immediate cause of death: (Approximate interval: onset to death)

    b. Due to or as a consequence of: (Interval: onset to death)

    c. Due to or as a consequence of: (Interval: onset to death)

    d. Due to or as a consequence of: (Interval: onset to death)

If I had filled out my father's death certificate, it would have read like this:

Immediate cause of death: dehydration (onset 4 days)

    a. Due to: dysphagia (onset 5 weeks)

    b. Due to: multiple lacunar infarcts (onset 6 months)

    c. Due to: coagulopathy (onset unknown)

    d. Due to: lymphoma (onset 8 years)

This document says that my father died after four days without food or fluid because it was deemed that his swallowing difficulty (dysphagia) was leading to dangerous choking. The swallowing difficulty was the result of multiple tiny strokes (lacunar infarcts). The strokes were caused by a clotting disorder (coagulopathy) that was a side effect of his lymphoma.[1]

What the distant observer can assume from this analysis is that the multiple strokes resulted in progressive disability over the last six months. One can further assume that somewhere between three and five days before his death, after discontinuation of food and fluid, Dad slipped into a coma and died comfortably.

One can also assume that his death was not sublimely serene; few are. It is important to note that over the last three weeks he received drops of morphine under the tongue to keep his breathing regular and a tranquilizer to keep any agitation at a minimum.

But more important for this exercise, it is what we did not do that allowed my father to progress to a quiet death. We did not pursue aggressive treatment for his lymphoma. We did not try to analyze and treat the causes of his mini-strokes. We did not start artificial hydration when his swallowing dysfunction made drinking unsafe.

REPRESENTATIVE DEATH CERTIFICATES

Now let's look at a series of hypothetical death certificates to make several points about the final act leading to the deathbed scene of several of the chronic illnesses described in chapter 5. The first certificate deals with lung cancer. It describes a patient who died ninety minutes after a blood clot to the lungs. The second certificate deals with heart failure. It describes a patient who died five minutes after the onset of ventricular fibrillation. The third certificate deals with cancer and liver failure from a disease of a disordered immune system. It describes a patient who died six days after slipping into a coma from liver failure.

Death Certificate #1

Immediate cause of death (other than cardiac arrest): Pulmonary embolus (onset ninety minutes)
    Due to: Thrombophlebitis (onset two weeks)
    Due to: Lung cancer (onset ten months)

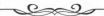

Death Certificate #2

Immediate cause of death (other than cardiac arrest): Ventricular fibrillation (onset five minutes)
>   Due to: Congestive heart failure (onset six years)
>   Due to: Cardiomyopathy (onset seven years)

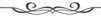

Death Certificate #3

Immediate cause of death (other than cardiac arrest): Hepatic coma (onset six days)
>   Due to: Bile duct cancer (onset one year)
>   Due to: Ulcerative colitis (onset twenty years)

By reviewing these documents we can better understand the sequence of events as outlined, the consequences of clinical decisions, and the factors that might lead to a more comfortable death.

Death Certificate #1: Working Backward

Death certificate #1 is about a hypothetical patient but it could have been my mother's. It lists pulmonary embolus (PE—a blood clot to the lungs) as the primary cause of death. In this scenario the heart and lungs probably stopped simultaneously resulting in a very quick passage from vital to non-vital, free of pulse and respirations. This patient would have lost consciousness within seconds of the final blood clot blocking flow.

I suspect that my mother might have passed away in this manner. It was either a PE from an unsuspected phlebitis or a cardiac arrhythmia.

Now, death by pulmonary embolus is a specific diagnosis that is not easily made clinically. It is generally made by some combination of X-ray studies.[2] Therefore, to accurately list that diagnosis, one can assume that this hypothetical patient died in the hospital. Consider what a hospitalization for a pulmonary embolus involves. Imagine the hustle and bustle of an ICU or cardiac ward: nurses, orderlies, and gurneys coming and going throughout the day and night; monitors beeping incessantly; multiple blood draws per day to monitor blood thinner therapy; and multiple urgent trips to radiology for tests. This is not a pretty scene. This is a stressful situation and an uncomfortable death—a necessary undertaking for young patients with a chance for a long reprieve but usually a mistake for elderly patients with an already foreshortened future.

So let's analyze this death certificate more closely, thinking about the course of illness and potential decision points where an aging patient might move toward a better death than that associated with aggressive therapy.

Death Certificate #1: Decision Points

At any time during the treatment of the lung cancer, when the oncologist says for the second or third time that "this combination of treatment is not working, we should consider changing course," the patient could exercise their option to cease aggressive therapy and enter a palliative care program or hospice care.

Whether the patient chooses that or not, the development of thrombophlebitis heralds a new level of illness. It suggests that the cancer is having widespread effects on the body, beyond immediate local effects on the lungs or bronchi. Proteins secreted by the tumor are circulating through the blood and have altered the delicately balanced clotting system. This is one example of what doctors call "systemic" effects. Whenever one of my patients exhibited a systemic effect of an apparently local cancer it proved to be a "poor prognostic indicator." That is doctor-speak (medical euphemism) for "your cancer is worse than we thought."

Again, when a new level of illness is recognized, a patient should re-evaluate aggressive hospitalized care. By going into the hospital to evaluate the swollen leg associated with blood clots in the veins, this hypothetical patient has re-engaged in the cycle of diagnosis and treatment from which it is so difficult to break free. At some point, the instinctive fear of death can be mitigated by the rational fear of a stressful, lonely, painful hospitalization. My mother, already in hospice care, would have stayed home in a similar situation and received palliative medications, oxygen, and morphine. These would have maximized her chances of a comfortable coma, and she would have avoided the futile treatments and the distress of a hectic hospital scene.

Death Certificate #2: Working Backward

Death certificate #2 documents a hypothetical cardiac death with some significant differences from the cancer-related death in the first example. Ventricular fibrillation is a rapid and painless way to expire, but it is a diagnosis that requires some electrocardiographic documentation to record with authority. This suggests the patient was in some monitored setting (ICU, ER, or ambulance) where the rhythm was recorded and unsuccessfully treated.

Backing up to the long-term diagnosis of congestive heart failure (see chapter 5) we should remind ourselves that this is the most common cause of death in the elderly. Its clinical course is marked by multiple doctor visits, hospitalizations, medication adjustments, and progressive decline. Many patients with advanced CHF will be candidates for mechanical interventions (pacemaker/defibrillators, heart valve replacements, left ventricular assist devices) and some will be candidates for heart transplant surgery.

Backing up further, we come to the diagnosis of cardiomyopathy, which means disease of the heart muscle. The most common cause of cardiomyopathy is atherosclerosis, the accumulation of fat and cholesterol, causing narrowed arteries, decreased blood flow, and decreased oxygenation of the muscle. Starved of oxygen, the muscle fibers die. The muscle death can involve large quantities of muscle during a single event (a heart attack or myocardial infarction), or individual fibers might die with an accumulation of problems over time.

Other causes of cardiomyopathy include viruses, deposition of abnormal proteins, and the toxic effects of medications, drugs, or alcohol. Each cause has variable prognostic implications. But the vast majority of heart muscle disease is progressive, and when it is, the downward spiral becomes observable and then predictable.

Death Certificate #2: Decision Points

Having worked backward to explore the disease pathways that point to this frequent cause of death, how could this patient and family have used an understanding of this disease to make decisions leading to a less medicalized death?

When a patient or family member recognizes a pattern of recurrent clinical events associated with congestive heart failure, a discussion should occur to determine how much longer to be aggressive and when to become passive. Recurrent episodes of water on the lungs (pulmonary edema), somnolence from low sodium (hyponatremia), and phlebitis predict future such events. Recurrent hospitalizations and doctor visits might lead to temporary improvement but ultimately lead to frustration as each treatment provides progressively less benefit. By the time a seventy-year-old patient has had their fourth hospitalization for heart failure or their second in a single month, their median life expectancy is six months.[3] Once this downward spiral is recognized, patients can make valid choices to intervene.

First and foremost, because of the poor results of cardiopulmonary resuscitation, elderly patients with chronic disease should consider establishing a Do Not Resuscitate (DNR) status. Patients living with the decline of advanced CHF can also indicate to their family and their doctors when to turn off their defibrillators, when to stop or decline dialysis, and when to stop potassium supplements and anticoagulants. All of these actions and inactions will promote quieter deaths by arrhythmia or coma. Patients can also decide how many episodes of pulmonary edema and pneumonia (a common fellow traveler) they want treated before requesting only morphine for comfort.

Death Certificate #3: Working Backward

This death certificate could have been filed for one of my most fascinating, complicated, memorable, and cherished patients, who suffered from two chronic illnesses that cause multiple problems when they occur together. She was an executive with a lobbying association in DC. She was referred to me for a change in bowel habits. I diagnosed ulcerative colitis and minor, nonspecific, changes in her liver function tests.

Ulcerative colitis is an inflammation of the colon that causes rectal bleeding, diarrhea, and cramping pain. Suppressing the immune system generally controls these symptoms. The mainstay of therapy at that time was steroids (prednisone-like medications) and with them her symptoms would be pushed into remission. Understandably, she did not enjoy the swelling and fluid retention that resulted from their use. Because her liver tests were mildly abnormal, the specter of a liver disease called sclerosing cholangitis loomed in the future. Ulcerative colitis and sclerosing cholangitis increase the lifetime risks of colon cancer and bile duct cancer, respectively. These facts, and her practical perspective on the ironies of life (for example, when her employment-sponsored insurance policy changed, she always searched for the plan with the best option for a liver transplant), allowed us to have many forward-looking, albeit pessimistic, conversations about advanced disease, worst-case scenarios, and end-of-life planning.

When biopsies of her colon showed widespread precancerous change, she subsequently had her colon removed. About that time her liver disease progressed. Despite second opinions and treatments with world-famous liver and bile duct specialists, her liver began to fail and a liver transplant was scheduled. Pathology on her resected liver found what pre-operative biopsies did not. She had cancer of the bile duct that was not completely removed with the surgery. This cancer, equal to pancreatic cancer in terms of dread outcomes, was made worse by the advanced immunosuppression required to retain her new liver.

When the bile duct cancer had consumed most of her new liver, she entered hospice care. Supported by her sister, she stopped fighting the cancer and allowed herself to slip into the coma of advanced liver failure.

Death Certificate #3: Decision Points

Although liver failure is not one of the six most common causes of death in the United States, it does exemplify the metabolic changes that lead to an altered mental status (think sleepiness or peaceful confusion) and coma which are common to many end-stage illnesses and which are quiet, painless, and comparatively quick ways to expire.

Patients with liver failure, kidney failure, or the metabolic disarray caused by untreated diabetes or dehydration can exercise the option of discontinuing supportive care, such as dialysis, at any time. Like the heart failure patient who recognizes the futility of repeated interventions, these patients can define a predetermined threshold or limit of interventions after which they will decline treatments or actively withdraw treatments. These patients can then pass their remaining time with the expectation that some arrhythmia or coma will allow them to slip away, hopefully peacefully. These decisions are frequently accompanied by a sense of empowerment and independence as one asserts one's will and individuality in the face of medical conformity and the momentum to treat.

Although the practice of medicine and the course of any disease process are predictably inexact, patterns can be recognized. Historically, attempts to influence those patterns are usually active treatment choices. When active treatment is likely to fail, yet cause more pain and disruption, then aggressively passive care is a better plan.

PNEUMONIA: COMMON TO MANY CHRONIC ILLNESSES

Now let us explore hypothetical examples of death certificates related to Alzheimer's disease, chronic lung disease, and stroke using a similar format but another jurisdiction's terminology:

Primary cause of death (other than cardiac arrest): _____
(onset, duration)
    Secondary to: _____(duration)
    Secondary to: _____(duration)

Death Certificate #4

Primary cause of death (other than cardiac arrest): Pneumonia (see date and time of death, one week)

    Secondary to: Aspiration (one week)

    Secondary to: Alzheimer's disease (eight years)

Death Certificate #5

Primary cause of death (other than cardiac arrest): Pneumonia (see date and time of death, one week)

    Secondary to: Emphysema (ten years)

    Secondary to: Tobacco addiction (fifty years)

Death Certificate #6

Primary cause of death (other than cardiac arrest): Pneumonia (see date and time of death, one week)

    Secondary to: Aspiration (two weeks)

    Secondary to: Stroke with dysphagia (six weeks)

What is common to these examples is that pneumonia is the ultimate cause of death in all three. If the lung cancer patient of example number one had not died of a pulmonary embolus and the heart failure patient of example number two had not died of ventricular fibrillation, there is a good chance that they would have (or did have) episodes of pneumonia. The short course described in each of the last three cases suggests that the infection was overwhelming or that antibiotics were declined and that the patients were made comfortable with morphine. Although aspiration pneumonia (the pneumonia caused by choking and breathing in bacteria) is common in debilitated patients, the pneumonia of COPD (chronic obstructive pulmonary disease) is also caused by the exacerbation of a chronic, already ongoing, infection.

SEPSIS—FRIEND OF THE AGED

By listing pneumonia as the cause of death on the preceding hypothetical death certificates, the presumption is that the patients died of respiratory failure. This means that their breathing became too shallow and labored to maintain adequate oxygen levels in the blood. The brain and the heart are most critically sensitive to oxygen deprivation. Low levels of oxygen lead to confusion, coma, heart rhythm disturbances, and (ultimately) cardiac arrest. As these organs fade, morphine keeps the patient relatively comfortable.

But pneumonia, like other bacterial infections, frequently causes death by another physiologic pathway, and that is sepsis.

Sepsis is the invasion of germs and toxins into the bloodstream that follows untreated bacterial infections. Doctors perceive of it as painless or "well tolerated" (doctor-speak for "comfortable enough") because it is a common cause of confusion or coma before evidence of an infection is manifest. For example, if an eighty-year-old woman arrives in the emergency room in a coma, the ER doctor has to run through the differential diagnosis appropriate to the circumstances. Usually a caregiver brings the patient in and gives a typical history, stating, "She was just fine a few hours ago, no complaints, not in pain, then she was a little confused, but when she stopped talking, I called 911." The ER doctor will check blood sugar, consider a drug overdose, check for evidence of a stroke, and so on, and when no other routine cause for coma is found, they will say to themselves, staff, and observers, "Sepsis can cause this—we had better check her out for an infection."[4]

Sticking with the example of that ER patient, it is important to emphasize that the process started without the patient's complaints and without the caregiver's observations of pain. No localizing symptoms rose to the level of concern. Maybe there was some coughing suggestive of pneumonia. Maybe there was urinary frequency, suggestive of a bladder infection. Whatever they were, these symptoms were mild enough to have gone unnoticed or to have been ignored. Every doctor in training will have experienced many cases of sepsis developing, painlessly, in hospitalized patients under their care for another problem.

Pneumonia and bladder infections are the most frequent and familiar infections, but many other infections can cause painless confusion and coma. Bedsores can lead to sepsis. In my years of practice, I saw dozens of patients with painless bile duct infections and the occasional patient with painless diverticulitis (an infection in the wall of the bowel) that led to sepsis.

Frequently, a comatose patient will be found to have bacteria in the blood, and no apparent source of the primary infection is ever found. That is idiopathic sepsis, which is considered by the CDC to be the tenth leading cause of death in the elderly.

Of course, some infections—such as abscesses—are painful. A painful infection should be palliated as needed with drainage, pain medications, and antibiotics—when necessary or desired. But the real point to take home is that painless infections will lead to sepsis and sepsis is a comparatively quick and comfortable way to die.

Therefore, it is important to include infections and ultimately sepsis in our vision of a comfortable death. Ezekiel Emanuel did so in his essay in *The Atlantic* when he stated that he would not take antibiotics after the age of seventy-five. He quotes Sir William Osler, the Johns Hopkins physician credited with founding modern medical education, who said, "Pneumonia may well be called the friend of the aged. Taken off by it in an acute, short, not often painful illness, the old man escapes those 'cold gradations of decay' so distressing to himself and to his friends."

Although Osler was unfamiliar with sepsis as we know it today, he designated pneumonia as the "friend of the aged" for multiple reasons. It is easy to diagnose. Its symptoms are easy to control with oxygen and morphine. It is comparatively comfortable. And, without treatment, it is usually fatal, either by respiratory failure or sepsis.

Most people will find Emanuel's seventy-fifth birthday an arbitrarily harsh line to draw. I certainly do. But when we, as individuals of an advanced age, recognize the arc of our decline, we should prepare to establish some guidelines for our family and ourselves.

EXIT STRATEGY

The point behind my exercise of reviewing death certificates is to look at the process from a different perspective. With chronic illnesses, there are some final commonalities and a few ways to expire more naturally (i.e., with less medical intervention), with some degree of control, and with minimal discomfort. When we stop trying to delay death with aggressive treatments and mechanical interventions, death is likely to come quietly from the coma of sepsis or dehydration—sometimes more quickly from a blood clot or an abnormal heart rhythm.

Creating a vision of such a death is the first step in avoiding endless, and frequently painful, treatment. The next step is to communicate that vision to your physicians, family, and friends. The final step is to accept that vision as an exit opportunity and perhaps work toward that vision as an exit strategy.[5] Sepsis, the respiratory failure of pneumonia (with morphine for comfort), a sudden arrhythmia, dehydration, low blood sugar, or a metabolically induced coma can be such an exit strategy.

If a patient and family can see a pattern of hospitalization, treatment, and diminished performance status repeat itself, that is a good time to discuss breaking that cycle. Choose hospice care. Identify treatments to be declined, such as antibiotics. Stop medications that prevent illness or prolong life. Turn off mechanical support devices such as pacemakers and defibrillators. Take medications for comfort. Decline doctor visits. Seek family visits. Aim for a coma. Visualize an exit option. Identify an exit strategy. These can be empowering choices that avoid medicalization and futile treatment.

One patient I spoke with had called me in to discuss the voluntary refusal of fluid and food. She was living a bed-to-chair existence and sleeping poorly because of urinary incontinence from multiple ministrokes. She was exhausted and ready to accept her mortality. Yet she was resisting the initial insertion of a bladder catheter as one indignity too far. The thought of such an invasion of her body, followed by routine catheter exchanges to prevent infection, brought tears to her eyes and a ripple of sadness across her face.

As planned, we discussed the death of dehydration by refusing to drink and eat. But she brightened in particular when I explained that inserting the catheter to avoid bedwetting would improve her sleep and decrease her fatigue. Subsequently refusing to exchange the catheter would ultimately create a urinary-tract infection, usually with minimal discomfort. If she chose, she could then decline antibiotics, and with the help of palliative medications she would be able to die comparatively comfortably of a progressive systemic infection. She now had a second exit strategy. She felt empowered, and her eyes twinkled.

Although the development of an exit strategy can precede a

terminal condition, the single most important step to implement a strategy is to seek hospice care. Before being admitted to hospice care, patients are subject to uncoordinated treatments from independent practitioners with goals that are not always in the patient's best interests. After being admitted to hospice care, the health care team is focused only on comfort and care. Working in what is effectively an alternate medical system, the doctors and nurses of the hospice care team offer individualized approaches to problems with the goal of preventing hospitalization and painful, stressful care with limited benefit. According to the National Hospice and Palliative Care Organization press releases, there are multiple studies showing that patients enrolled in hospice, especially home hospice, live slightly longer than similar patients undergoing hospital treatments. And while comfort care measures do not guarantee, but do maximize the possibility of, a quiet death, the alternative—endlessly seeking treatment—virtually guarantees painful medicalization without a real promise of long-term benefit. More about hospice care in chapter 11.

Things to Remember/Things to Consider

- Discuss with your doctor what they foresee as likely causes of death given your diagnosis: pneumonia, respiratory failure, or hemorrhage, for example.
- Create a vision of where that death might best occur.
- Share your vision with friends, family, and physicians.
- Consider an exit strategy—an illness for which you will decline treatment.
- When aggressive treatment results in complications and limited benefit, consider passive care, then hospice care, and then an exit opportunity.

Chapter Seven

Dad's Final Weeks

Man, as long as he lives, is immortal. One minute before his death he shall be immortal. But one minute later, God wins.
—Elie Wiesel

B ELYING THE ACCURACY of the death certificates described in the last chapter (including the hypothetical example that I offered of my father's), Dad's actual death certificate was a work of stunning simplicity. It read, "Immediate cause of death: Lymphoma—Interval between onset and death: 8 years." This document is grossly inadequate for a hospitalized death, but the coroner and other authorities tolerated this simplicity because he died in hospice care. Hospice nurses documented his decline in their official records, and his admission to hospice care certified that his death would not be either unexpected or suspicious.

Similarly, the scene surrounding my father's death was not dramatic, but death is never simple. The notebooks used by his caregivers to communicate among themselves document the daily struggle to deal with his symptoms of fatigue and constant itching as well as the challenges of keeping debilitated patients clean and dying patients comfortable.[1] The caregiver team my sisters put together was exceptionally good in every regard.

Dad died as he had declined, a gradual loss of functional ability over several years until an accelerated deterioration at the very end.

In retrospect, the last chapter began on the eve of his final Christmas. It ended four months later on April twenty-fifth.

My wife, Debbie, and I visited him over Christmas. It was a hastily planned trip as the reality of the holidays arrived. Since September my sisters and I had been rotating our visits with increasing frequency, but we had not focused on the holidays. This would be the first Christmas when he was too weak to visit friends and neighbors, so it fell to us to entertain him.

Debbie and I shared the goal of bringing back some old Christmas memories. I had another goal. I wanted to reopen talks about exit strategies. I knew he was interested, but following his admission to home hospice he seemed to have achieved a new plateau of physical and emotional stability. It seemed that he could now go on forever with twenty-four–seven coverage by health aides, domestic staff, and nursing personnel, taking three meals a day at the table and spending the other twenty-two hours per day in bed while listening to audio books and news reports.

In September, Dad and I had discussed discontinuing his routine medications. No action had been taken, primarily because no predictable result would occur. No specific medication was keeping him alive (such as insulin) so no specific outcome could be foreseen. But Dad wanted to revisit the medication list as a potential exit strategy. On December twenty-fourth we discussed it again. I advised him that I supported the idea in principle, particularly because there had been subtle, but progressive, swallowing difficulties. Other than less choking with pills at breakfast, I reminded him that the decision was largely symbolic, and no specific outcome could be predicted.

We also repeated the discussion about the voluntary refusal of fluid and food as an exit strategy. This conversation took on the familiar circularity of previous discussions. His appetite remained strong, and his meals gave him pleasure. They were a major focus of each day and remained so until his final days. In fact, one of the last sentences he spoke, and one of the last requests he made, occurred months later during his final breakfast. He sent his last English muffin back for more butter and more English marmalade.

"Starvation is not an exit strategy for me," he repeated in December and again in January.

"Dad, it is not starvation, it is dehydration. And anyway, that means you are not yet ready to consider the option now, but when you are ready, you will know it," I responded, yet again.

We left the evening of Christmas Day to visit our West Coast children. On December twenty-sixth, Dad called the nurse managing his caregivers and advised her that he would not be taking any more routine medications. He would take pain pills and medications directed at specific symptoms (his steroids for itching, for example). He called his hospice nurse and advised her there was no need to refill his heart, blood pressure, cholesterol, or depression pills. He sent an email to his children advising us of this decision. If nothing else, it signaled that he was getting ready for the inevitable in his own way.

I visited a month later. Clinical changes were subtle. His mind remained sharp but his manual dexterity, as evidenced by dropping food at the table, was worse. The following month his legs nearly collapsed beneath him as he was transferring from the bed to the wheelchair. In retrospect, I think this was the result of another mini-stroke. Now he could no longer transfer safely with just one assistant to guide him.

A NURSING ASSISTANT'S REVELATION

Following his dramatic leg weakness and the near fall while transfer-ring, an event that occurred the day before my last visit, we promptly acquired a "Get-U-Up" hoist (I did not make that name up) from the hospice. It arrived within a day. But hoists are complicated, and each of his caregivers had to be trained in its use. Like so many elderly patients my father was very anxious about being suspended in a sling. I hopefully assumed he would get used to it in a short time.

My sisters and I thought we would settle into another new normal. We trusted that because he had lived for five months with full-time assistance from bed to chair and commode transfers, then he would settle into a new pace of transfers with the hoist.

Before the hoist, he was out of bed five or six times per day (three meals at the dining room table, a cocktail in the living room every eve-ning, and the sometime trip to the building's deck or lobby). After the hoist's arrival, we figured that we would schedule a morning transfer with the hoist and two staff, coupling that with his morning bathing. Then it would be lunch in bed and perhaps an evening transfer, up for dinner at the table, and then back to bed with a commode stop along the way. We assumed this new normal could go on for months.

But two things happened that changed that outlook. First, Dad hated the hoist so much that he ordered it removed within days of my departure. He was now bed-bound.

Second, and shortly thereafter, a Certified Nursing Assistant who had performed his bed baths for months took my older sister—newly arrived for a long stay—aside. She explained that in her experience, when a formerly modest man became unconcerned about modesty, he usually died within a month. She then noted that Dad did not express concern about a new nurse trainee that day. Her countdown had begun.

I doubted the importance or validity of this observation. But, in fact, Dad died three weeks later.

My father's involuntary decline in oral intake of food and fluid accelerated at that point. It paralleled other deterioration. He was becoming even sleepier. His arms were becoming weaker and stiffer. His swallowing was progressively problematic. Gently encouraging food and drink was making him anxious and frustrated. His advance directive included a clause that eliminated spoon feeding if there was no reasonable hope for improvement. It was his experienced staff that announced they were uncomfortable feeding him. They determined that his swallowing was dangerously ineffective. He was choking regularly. Despite having adamantly refused to voluntarily discontinue food and fluid prior to this point, he did not complain or ask for spoon feeding to be continued.

During his last week, he began to move in and out of consciousness. Occasionally, he called out for someone, including his mother, or muttered nonsensically. The hospice nurses described this state as "actively dying."[2] When my father achieved this state of altered mental status, we knew that he would die without pain. But we did not know how long he would last. His caregivers were documenting a pattern of irregular breathing. There were periods of rapid breaths, slow breaths, and progressively long pauses between episodes of rapid breathing. Morphine and tranquilizers were being adjusted regularly to regulate breathing, comfort, and agitation.

My sister and I were having regular conversations at this point. Dad had effectively given up food and fluid. What little he consumed in the days before was not enough to sustain him but might have been enough to prolong the process. I reminded my sister that when patients voluntarily refused food and fluid, 85 percent were dead within two weeks.[3] But this fact did not offer true comfort. We did not know exactly when his "two week" period started. More important, 15 percent were alive at two weeks, and the rare patient survived six weeks without food or fluid.

He could have died any moment, but he might have hung on. We could only comfort ourselves by reassuring each other that he was being kept clean and comfortable. Fortunately, he died five days after his last sip of fluid and his last bite of food. My sister was there for him and for us.

FINAL THOUGHTS

The moment of my father's death emphasizes the insignificance of distinguishing between cardiac arrest and respiratory arrest. During his last weeks the hospice nurses had been visiting on a daily basis. They would take his vital signs and then discuss his physical needs with the staff. They answered questions and offered emotional support to my sister. On their very last visit, at his last hour, the first nurse came out of the bedroom to report to my sister that his blood pressure was good, his pulse was regular, and that his breathing was quiet. It appeared that he would live another day. Before the first nurse finished her report, the second nurse emerged and told my sister, "He has just passed away."

Of course, we were saddened by the news, but we were relieved. He was ready. We were ready. He had not suffered.

We were also relieved because there is no guarantee of success with this aggressively passive approach. Mistakes happen. Unexpected and frightening symptoms (seizures, hallucinations, uncontrollable pain, for example) can occur. Medicalization happens. Even under the best of circumstances the process of dying is messy, intense, unappealing, and unpredictable. But for my father, the process worked. His death was peaceful.

THE DEVELOPMENT OF HIS VISION

My father had witnessed several deathbed scenes during his lifetime. He had a client who died from complications of an aortic aneurysm. These facts informed his personal perspective.

Of course, he had observed his wife's death.

I also know that he had been attentive to sick friends, colleagues, and clients. I remember as a young teen when my father took me to visit a business associate who was dying of prostate cancer. I do not remember why we stopped for that visit. Dad and I were running errands, and he made the decision to visit and bring me along. I do remember the man, propped in bed and smelling of urine and impending doom.

On one of my trips, Dad described his last visit to the deathbed of his uncle John. "He was curled up in a fetal position. I was trying to probe his memory of his parents." That scene, as he described it, was eerily similar to what I was experiencing on my recent visits. Ultimately, Uncle John just slipped away.

The most poignant deathbed scene he described to me took place in about 1930. Dad was eight or nine years old. His grandfather, known as Pop, was dying at home. He was described as yellow, bloated, and swollen. It was probably pancreatic cancer with liver metastases and jaundice. Pop, a faithful Catholic, was distressed that his son had failed to raise my father in the Catholic religion. On this occasion, Pop had asked to see my father, alone. Pop pressed his rosary into his grandson's hand. Dad left with his secret new possession. Pop died quietly soon thereafter.

Finally, I note that my father had been through World War II as a naval officer with Japanese language skills. He landed with the army on Kwajelein and Okinawa. He transported Japanese POWs from Okinawa to Hawaii. Many of those POWs died of tetanus. Others

died from internecine fighting between the Japanese and the Oki-
nawans. As a translator, my father served on the team that intervened
in these matters. Dad had seen death. Perhaps he had witnessed or
experienced periods of hunger.

The point of these reflections is to note that, unlike so many, Dad
knew about death and dying. He grew up in the era when people died
at home. He had seen it. He knew it could be natural, without excessive
medical interventions. From his war years he learned it could be unnatural and unfair. Toughened to those realities, he was able to cope.

THE INFLUENCE OF PAIN

My father was gracious and kind to the end. He faced his decline with
courage and equanimity. With respect to pain, however, my father
was not particularly courageous. He tolerated pain stoically but certainly not heroically. Fortunately, during his last eight years, we were
never really challenged. He suffered only three episodes of acute pain
syndromes. Two episodes were related to otherwise minor falls that
resulted in tiny cracks in his vertebrae.[4] A third episode was that of
a torn hamstring that was a complication of his physical therapy
program.

When present, chronic pain saps the strength of almost everyone.
It changes grief to depression and depression to despair. I am confident
that my father's experiences with the Great Depression, the Second
World War, and his unwaveringly good appetite molded his perspective on hastening death by refusing to eat and drink. I am equally confident that if he had suffered an open-ended, chronic pain condition
he would have found giving up fluid and food a satisfactory way to
expedite the process.

My father began many of our conversations by saying, "I never knew how hard it would be to die." But doing it the way he did allowed us to let go gracefully. Finally, peace had arrived.

Things to Remember/Things to Consider

- Good caregivers are essential.
- Hospice professionals have many insights to offer.
- "Actively dying" creates symptoms that are poorly understood.
- Difficulty managing pain might alter a patient's perspective on hastening their death.
- Discontinuing routine medications is one technique that might shorten the dying process.

Chapter Eight

How to Recognize a Terminal Diagnosis

I am not afraid to die. I just don't want to be there when it happens.

—Woody Allen

———

WHEN FORMER PRESIDENT Jimmy Carter announced in the summer of 2015 that he had metastatic melanoma, I judged immediately that he had a terminal diagnosis. I did not know how long he would live, what treatment he would choose, or when he would die, but I understood that he would eventually die of melanoma or with melanoma. As I write this book, he is in remission. He has enjoyed an excellent response to surgery, stereotactic radiation therapy, and immunotherapy. But that doesn't change the fact that his life will end as a result of melanoma, a complication of its treatment, or of old age with melanoma smoldering in remission or staging a relapse. His comments on his disease have expressed an understanding of his situation and an appreciation for his good response.

Unfortunately, most people do not share this same understanding. There is enormous resistance to recognizing a terminal illness and even greater resistance when the end is near. Most patients never want to face that prospect, most families are unwilling to address it, and most doctors are loath to broach the subject.

That is because "terminal" is a loaded term. Health care professionals avoid it because it inspires misinterpretation and misunderstanding. Family members avoid it because they think they are dooming the patient to an immediate hopelessness and flogging their awareness of imminent death by using it. Even health care organizations, government regulations, and end-of-life groups replace terminal illness with "serious" or "life-threatening" illness in their written publications to avoid the baggage.

When doctors say "terminal," patients usually hear "hopeless," infer immediacy, withdraw inward, and stop communicating. Arguably, when used alone, as in "his situation is terminal," this meaning applies. For these reasons, health care professionals and family members avoid it for as long as possible, and this only serves to enhance the negative power of the word.

For the purposes of this chapter, when I write "terminal illness" (disease or diagnosis), I'm referring to the specific illness that will likely be the cause of death without specifying a time frame for that process. Similarly, I use the phrase "terminal condition" or "situation" to indicate death is imminent (median life expectancy less than or equal to six months) from any cause. This chapter focuses on how to recognize both a terminal illness, such as cancer, nonmalignant chronic illness, and old age, and how it transitions into a terminal condition.

To be clear, having a terminal disease does not mean it is time to "give up." Recognizing a terminal diagnosis is different from surrendering to a terminal situation, but it is the first step toward accepting that ultimate development. Acknowledging a terminal disease, illness, or diagnosis allows one to study it, analyze its context, observe its course, and plan for the future. It does not preclude aggressive therapy.

But, within this framework, a patient or health care proxy can see the transition from a terminal illness to a terminal condition, and they can change the treatment plan accordingly. To foresee the terminal condition is to know the "why" and allows one to make the choices that influence the "where" and "when" of death.

In previous chapters I have attempted to simplify medical terminology and after an initial definition I have tried to minimize repeated uses of distracting medical terms. In this chapter I am going to try to translate medical terms and doctor-speak that are used to avoid the hard truth in end-of-life situations.

THE LESSONS OF ALS: DEALING WITH THE REALITY OF A TERMINAL ILLNESS

Loath as we Americans are to acknowledge a terminal diagnosis, there is one disease that we instantly recognize as such. That is amyotrophic lateral sclerosis (Lou Gehrig's disease), a disease that steals the physical strength from people of all ages without affecting their mental capacity. Exactly how this single disease acquired and maintains its recognizably terminal status is unclear. I suspect the fundamental reason is that there is no advertising campaign about treatment advances to mislead the public. As an orphan illness (one that affects only a small number of patients) there is less potential profit to be made from commercializing small treatment advances, so the public is largely unaware of any progress.

This is the opposite situation with cancer therapy, where we are bombarded with information about "progress." Witness the advertising campaigns supporting small advances with lung cancer.

Another factor might be that doctors are more honest with ALS patients. Having so little to offer in terms of treatment and nowhere to hide in terms of false hope, doctors and patients simply must learn to cope.

There is a lesson to be drawn from this. People can receive a terminal diagnosis and deal with it when they have to—because they have to.

During my career, I helped with several ALS patients. I was usually tasked with inserting and maintaining their feeding tubes. This offered me a window into the lives of patients who recognized they had a terminal illness and still managed to cope.

The slow-motion catastrophe of ALS is a compelling example of how the trajectory of an illness can be predicted. There tends to be a linear, downhill course with a median survival of three to five years. Charting the course of ALS is particularly easy by observing the functional loss of the arms and legs and by measuring the breathing capacity as a function of the weakening respiratory muscles. Because people know what is coming, because they are aware of the inevitable course of their illness, they are forced to plan. They are forced to make difficult decisions.

Of course, the biggest decision to be considered is whether or not to be placed on a breathing machine. Those patients who decline to be placed on a ventilator will die of respiratory failure. Those who do choose mechanical ventilation live for months or years bed-bound and chained to a machine. They die of a complication related to those conditions, usually an infection with an antibiotic-resistant bacteria.

Ninety percent of ALS patients ultimately refuse mechanical ventilation. One important factor in this decision is financial—it is the rare patient that has insurance coverage for long-term ventilatory support. But more important, knowing they have a terminal illness and living its slow-motion ravages, they have to deal with reality and cannot hide behind a hypothetical. They have time to consider the consequences of their decisions and with the aid of support groups are able to observe other ALS patients both with and without mechanical ventilation.

In my community, a friend and neighbor was diagnosed with ALS in his early sixties. Within two years his disability was so advanced that he was effectively homebound and almost bed-bound. He and his wife decided against mechanical ventilation because they saw the families clinging to life torn apart by their dependency on the machines. An artist, he changed his subject matter from landscapes to portraits as his disease progressed. Too weak to grip a paintbrush, his assistants strapped the brushes to his arms, torso, or head. With coarse strokes and within a limited range he crafted portraits of his neighbors at a pace of almost one per day. During the last eight months of his life, in a flurry of artistic activity, he devoted his efforts to enhancing his legacy rather than clinging to life. Enormously brave, he used the recognition of his terminal condition to his advantage. Aided by palliative medications, he died quietly of respiratory failure, in his sleep, his wife at his side.

RECOGNIZING TERMINAL CANCER

Most family members feel too constrained by sensitivity issues to introduce a discussion of the topic of a terminal illness—if they can bring themselves to think about it at all. "Why bring it up before we have to?" is the frequently unasked question all parties embrace. As long as we can cling to the false promise of a cure we don't have to deal with terminal truth. Yet in my experience, every patient with a diagnosis of advanced cancer has thought about the terminal nature of his or her illness, and most are willing to discuss it long before their doctors and family members are. Those who acknowledge it early can use the power of the diagnosis to their advantage—just as my friend with ALS did.

How can you recognize a terminal illness before being shocked by the conclusion that you have a terminal condition? First, let us start with the obvious. Many cancers are treatable but incurable. Most of us know this, but refuse to acknowledge it. Our tendency is to deny a terminal diagnosis and to embrace the hope of a cure. When we see a headline such as "Precision Cancer Therapy Promises Paradigm Shift," we prefer to believe we are winning the "war on cancer" rather than struggle with the uncomfortable truth that victory is a long way off.[1]

One way to recognize an illness that is likely to become terminal is to understand when certain terms such as "metastatic," "stage II," or "advanced" are used to qualify the cancer diagnosis. Metastatic means that the cancer has spread beyond the confines of the original organ. Stages of cancer describe how far the metastases have spread. There are many staging algorithms, but in broad terms: stage 0 means superficial cancer; stage I means cancer limited to the organ of origin; stage II means the cancer has spread to adjacent tissues or organs; Stage III means extensive local spread with lymph node involvement; and stage IV means widespread or distant metastases.[2] When a doctor says "advanced" cancer, they mean metastatic or greater than stage I. In general, widespread, advanced, or stage III and above cancers will prove to be terminal. There are exceptions to this rule, but it is better to be pleasantly surprised than hopelessly Pollyannaish.

In reality, most advanced cancers of the brain, pancreas, lung, liver, bile duct, stomach, intestines, ovaries, and melanoma are ultimately going to carry the patient away unless the initial surgery is brilliantly successful, leaving no traces of cancer behind. If tumor is left behind, or if the patient is deemed not to be a surgical candidate—one whose tumor has already spread or one who is too weak to survive surgery—then it is the very rare patient who gets indefinite benefit from the blocking tactics of radiation and chemotherapy.

This is not to say that an elderly patient, on receipt of such a diagnosis, should simply "curl up and die" (although a major goal of this book is to remind you when to exercise the option to decline treatment); but when a patient is given one of these diagnoses, they should exercise judgment about the medical advice they receive as to how aggressively to treat and for how long.

Anyone over sixty-five with evidence of a chronic illness falls into this category. Anyone over the average life expectancy for their demographic should also think long and hard about any intervention for one of these advanced cancers, because palliative care might offer a longer life expectancy in addition to a better quality of life than aggressive treatment. But if "young" and brave, or if the pre-op scans look promising, try for curative surgery. Try a course of chemotherapy, but carefully weigh the side effects versus the measurable benefits.

When my mother was told she had stage IV non–small cell carcinoma of the lung, neither she nor my father heard that she had a terminal illness, but that was the fact. When oncologists say "stage IV" or "end-stage" anything, they are skirting the "terminal" issue and inviting patients to gloss over it. Most likely, the oncologist did not emphasize those specific words, and if he did, their meaning was successfully sidestepped. My parents knew it was serious; both had listened closely. Yet at first blush they failed to grasp the fact that Mom would ultimately die of lung cancer if she did not die of something else sooner.

I suspect my mother recognized her condition as terminal before my father did. This is partly because of the dynamics of a caring couple. The sick member of a pair will see his or her condition from the glass-half-empty perspective but will convince him or herself to survive for the benefit of the other. The well member of the pair will see the illness from the glass-half-full perspective and will vow to help with the "cure."

In my mother's case, I think she understood her condition before my father did because she was without pretense or self-importance. She had worked for years as a pediatric nurse, so from a health care perspective, she knew that disease happened. Earlier in life, she had nursed friends and family members on their deathbeds. However, she could not verbalize the terminal nature of her condition until I did it for her.

STANDARDIZED TREATMENTS

After receiving a diagnosis of cancer, the first question people often ask is, "How could this happen to me?" The second question is, "Where is the best treatment?" In truth, chemotherapeutic protocols are standardized across the spectrum of academic and commercial oncology programs. Not only is the cure not just over the horizon in a temporal sense; it isn't just around the corner in a physical sense, either. With the exception of particularly rare cancers, where one center might have more experience than another, there is little point in hoping that the cure will be found at another center. Cancer centers may vary in several respects, including the amenities they offer, but in this age of rapid dissemination of medical knowledge, no center is going to have a miraculous treatment for a common cancer that is unavailable to another.[3]

Chemotherapeutic protocols are not only standardized; they are ranked and utilized in a sequence that optimizes the benefits and minimizes the side effects. Therefore, one can conclude that the first-line treatment is the most effective and balanced with an acceptable level of complications. Subsequent treatments will be less effective and will generally have more side effects or complications. If your oncologist is offering you a second or third course of treatment, you are buying less time and at greater physical cost. If they are offering you a fourth or fifth type of chemotherapy, you should consider that your terminal illness is progressing to the terminal condition and you should make decisions accordingly.

NAILING COFFINS SHUT: ONCOLOGY, PALLIATIVE CARE, AND THE CONVERSATION

Conventionally trained oncologists are particularly loath to discuss the terminal aspect of a cancer under treatment. That's because it is their business and profession to treat, to offer treatment, to promote treatment and, in many cases, to overtreat. Oncologists treating the terminally ill often use euphemisms such as "hopefully," "buy some time," "have some benefit," "we can expect significant reduction in tumor burden," and "if this doesn't work, we can always try..." These are all ways of avoiding the truth—that this disease is incurable, and that the next course of chemotherapy, while not offering a cure, might even harm you. At an old age, not understanding these euphemisms frequently results in overexpectation and unwanted, painful overtreatment.

A friend recently told me about her eighty-nine-year-old mother's consultation with an oncologist for a newly diagnosed stage IV cancer of the pancreas. It serves as an example of this traditional, but not always helpful, dynamic.

After greeting her optimistically, the doctor immediately launched into a description of treatment options. The elderly woman listened and then posed the question, "At my age, how long can I expect to live if I decline chemotherapy, and how much longer can I expect to live if I undertake therapy?" When the doctor responded that the answer to both questions was three to six months, the elderly patient wisely paused to think. She was quite taken aback by the emphasis on treatment and ultimately declined aggressive therapy.

According to the science behind the studies, three months of added life expectancy with this disease is considered statistically significant, and the oncologist was trained to present it as such. But for many people at an advanced age, three months of added "life" in hospitals or nursing homes, while suffering side effects, is not an appealing prospect. Rather, it is a zero sum game. My friend's mother saw through the statistics and saw no practical benefit.

When I began my career, long before I became conscious of the limitations of modern medicine and while still a starry-eyed gastroenterologist with the best new résumé on the staff, I was asked to see a patient for a second opinion. The elderly gentleman had metastatic stomach cancer that had caused a partial blockage of the outlet of his stomach. The initial consulting gastroenterologist, a highly regarded member of the medical staff, had made aggressive recommendations consistent with the consulting oncologist's treatment plans. The family was unwilling to consider standard surgery to bypass the blockage and insert a feeding tube. The senior gastroenterologist was suggesting that my endoscopic technique for inserting a feeding tube and a second drainage tube would replace standard surgery and allow for future courses of chemotherapy. I was called in by the patient's family practitioner with the expectation that I would endorse those plans. I sensed an unspoken ambivalence on the part of the patient, the family, and the primary care practitioner. I also felt that the proposed treatment was not only too aggressive, but very likely to result in a complication.

As a result of my opinion, the patient and family chose to seek palliative care. Subsequently, while discussing the situation with the devoted family practitioner, I asked why the oncologist wanted to be so aggressive. His answer was this: "Sam, do you know why they nail coffins shut?" He waited a beat before giving away the punch line: "To keep the oncologists out."

Indeed, family practitioners or primary care internists are probably better than oncologists when trying to convey the terminal nature of a cancer. If their sympathetic personas are tempered with a dose of reality, you might hear the unvarnished truth. But some primary care physicians can be too closely attached to their patients, and their friendship might influence their judgment. These physicians may be too sympathetic and collude with family members to obscure the facts. It's important to be aware of this dynamic.

In the previous anecdote, there were two reasons the family practitioner asked my opinion. The first was to consider endorsing the aggressive gastrointestinal care needed to support the chemotherapy. If indeed it was the unanimous opinion to proceed, this would protect against subsequent complaints if complications arose. The second reason was to get an objective outsider's analysis. An objective outsider is more likely to make a hard-nosed calculation, uncluttered by emotion, and more likely to introduce the discussion of a terminal illness or terminal condition. This is a variation on an end-of-life discussion that has recently become known as "The Conversation" or "The Hard Conversation." I will discuss that in detail in chapter 10.

Not all oncologists are grave robbers. Most oncologists today are more conscious of palliative and hospice care than in the past, perhaps because in this day and age, some are board certified in both cancer therapy and palliative care. Seeking out such a physician is probably worthwhile. In any event, understanding an oncologist's perspective and track record on end-of-life issues before starting a treatment course with them is extremely important, as is a palliative care consult if the oncologist is not board certified in both disciplines. Unfortunately, most patients don't take the time to do this.

THE HARDEST CONVERSATION COMES HOME TO MY NEIGHBORHOOD

As a neighbor and a friend, I knew Sally well. Sally came to me in her early fifties with a vague stomach pain that had many qualities of a gastric ulcer. She was also suffering from neurological symptoms, including double vision, muscle weakness, and tingling in her extremities. By the time I saw her, her internist, an oncologist, and two neurologists had performed body scans, brain scans, and every type of mammogram (routine, MRI, ultrasound).

The possibility of a widespread cancer had been considered and was rejected when no lung, brain, pancreatic, ovarian, or breast cancer was identified on any scan. Further complicating her case was a remote history of mania that cast the specter of a psychiatric component over her otherwise inexplicable symptomatology. Referred by a distinguished and aggressive oncologist, she set aside her concerns about privacy and set up an appointment. As a physician, I interpreted the fact that she screwed up her courage to come see me as objective evidence that her symptoms were not psychiatric. It meant she was serious and seriously worried.

I advised Sally that a gastroscopy (an endoscopic examination of the stomach) was appropriate to exclude a small gastric ulcer. If benign, such an ulcer would only explain her belly pain. If malignant, such an ulcer might contribute to the understanding of her symptoms, but it would be very rare to have such an ulcer go unseen on her exams to date.

The scope exam of her stomach was uneventful, and the results appeared normal until the pathologist called me about the routine biopsies I had performed. He asked me if Sally had a known case of breast cancer. When I replied "No," he explained that he had found microscopic deposits of breast cancer, proven by special laboratory tests, scattered throughout the stomach tissue. An advanced form of breast cancer can look like this—billions of tiny implants of small numbers of cells scattered throughout different organs. In my limited experience, this manifestation usually occurred after more common presentations had been treated and further along in the course of the illness. In her case, the disease had spread before it could be detected by any standard means.

It suddenly became clear that Sally's neurological symptoms were related to microscopic, malignant implants in her nervous system. It was clear that the disease was far advanced and would be the cause of her death. Calling her in to discuss this completely unexpected finding of widely metastatic breast cancer in the face of negative mammograms was a surreal experience and a very difficult conversation.

Although it was clear that the disease would prove to be terminal, it was equally clear that the immediate situation was not yet a terminal condition. She was a young woman with high school– and college-aged children. In light of her youth, it was appropriate to emphasize treatment options optimistically. Although I did not mince words, it would have been inappropriate to overemphasize the "terminal" aspect at the time of her stunning diagnosis. Instead, we focused on the extraordinary circumstances of her presentation and how to manage the disease going forward.

But two and a half years later, when her follow-up chemotherapy stopped working, it was worth her remembering that she had a terminal diagnosis. She had done well with hormonal treatment and subsequent chemotherapy, but eventually she suffered the inevitable relapse. She now found herself with a truly terminal condition. Her oncologist had wanted to invoke one last heroic treatment. In agreement with her children that she had suffered enough, and without the promise of measurable benefit, she decided against it and had a comparatively quiet death.

CANCER PLUS A SECOND CHRONIC ILLNESS

Having a "poor prognosis" is a euphemism for having a terminal illness that is moving toward a terminal condition. For example, a cancer diagnosis combined with another system-wide or chronic illness is a poor prognostic indicator. This second disease is known as a comorbid condition. An example of this would be the diagnosis of lung cancer in a smoker with chronic lung disease or congestive heart failure.

An elderly patient should question the oncologist closely if he or she hears that the treatment options are limited by a comorbid disease. The implication is that the patient will not do as well as expected in established treatment algorithms or be a candidate for ongoing studies of new protocols.

Cancer trials (medical studies focused on emerging treatments) are performed on highly selected patients. Because researchers want to get the purest evaluation, not to mention the most promising results, from their trials, patients with complicated circumstances or comorbid illnesses that would complicate the analysis of a given treatment are excluded from participation. Therefore, if a cancer patient has a comorbid condition and doesn't fit the profile of the prior study group, they can expect that their chances of benefit will be reduced compared with the official results.

Similarly, if an oncologist offers to treat a patient outside of a new protocol, the patient should recognize that the benefits described by the protocol do not apply to them. The patient may choose to proceed but they should understand that they're likely to fare worse than the protocol average.

Another indicator of a poor prognosis is the presence of a widespread symptom caused by a local cancer. I referred to this in chapter 6 as "systemic effects" but it is technically referred to as a paraneoplastic condition. Nerve damage (neuropathy) is a common example of a paraneoplastic process. Although X-rays might show what appears to be a local tumor (limited to a single site within a single organ), the presence of the neuropathy indicates that some aspect of the cancer, usually an antibody but occasionally tumor cells, is circulating in the body and damaging tissue elsewhere. Chemotherapy might improve the neuropathy, but in my experience most patients with any paraneoplastic syndrome have a worse prognosis than patients with the same cancer but without the paraneoplastic process.

An example of this relates to a friend and neighbor. At age sixty-three he developed a painful burning of his hands and feet. The initial diagnosis was peripheral painful neuropathy of unclear origin. Sometimes a neuropathy just happens. Sometimes it is caused by another illness. Months passed as local physicians failed to make a primary diagnosis and were unable to adequately control the pain. Frustration mounted. Finally a third neurological consultation found a small lung cancer. As is frequently the case, despite its small size it was deemed inoperable, and a course of chemotherapy was undertaken with the goal of reducing the painful condition. Unfortunately, the pain persisted. My friend recognized that his prognosis was poor and the quality of his life was deteriorating. He entered hospice care and passed away more comfortably than if he had pursued further aggressive treatment.

NONMALIGNANT TERMINAL ILLNESSES

Certain combinations of non-cancer diagnoses, when added together, result in a terminal condition. The previous example from chapter 5 of John, diagnosed with heart disease, kidney failure, and diabetes, falls into this category. Of course, advanced age is to be factored in. Taken individually, each diagnosis can be manageable, but the sum of their various manifestations may be terminal. Doctors conflate these diseases into the catchall phrase "multisystem failure."

Recognizing a terminal diagnosis without the benefit of a malignant component can be difficult. We shudder when a doctor says "cancer." "Could this be the end?" we ask. But when a doctor says "end-stage heart disease" or "significant dementia" we think, "This sounds manageable; at least it's not cancer." The facts are different.

Advanced cases of chronic heart disease, chronic lung disease, chronic liver disease, and dementia are not malignant disorders but can be quantified and determined to be terminal. If your primary care physician will not help you research what defines the six-month median survival for your particular condition, ask to be referred to a geriatrician or palliative care specialist who will. Let me give you some examples of clinical scenarios where aggressive care is likely to be counterproductive at a minimum and possibly cruel.

As I mentioned in chapter 6, when a patient with advanced heart failure is seventy years or older, has had four hospitalizations for heart failure overall or a repeat hospitalization for heart failure within two months, and is dependent on others for three or more activities of daily living, then his or her median survival is less than six months, no matter what treatments are tried.

Therefore, one can infer from the previous statement that if a seventy-five-year-old patient is already working on his or her third hospitalization for heart failure, has very poor cardiac pumping ability, and is dependent on family or friends for bathing and dressing, then a personal Rubicon is approaching.

Or consider chronic obstructive pulmonary disease (COPD). If a patient is over the age of seventy, requires supplemental oxygen, has heart failure caused by the lung disease, has a Karnofsky Performance Status less than sixty (unable to work, requires considerable assistance with ADLs, requires frequent medical care), and shows evidence of malnutrition or kidney disease, then it is very unlikely that aggressive therapy will increase their life expectancy.[4]

These patients have decisions to make about how aggressively to pursue soon-to-be ineffective treatment or how aggressively to be passive, ultimately seeking palliation.

This type of calculation and projection can be applied to all cancers and major chronic illnesses, if you are willing to look into it.[5] A good geriatrician or an expert in palliative care can help analyze these data and appropriately place a patient on the end-of-life spectrum.

WHEN OLD AGE IS TERMINAL

"Geriatric failure to thrive" is one medical expression used for "dying of old age." The government bureaucrat's term for the same process is "the non-disease-specific decline in clinical status." When does one know that the terminal phase of old age is at hand? One certain guide is to study the Medicare requirements for admission to hospice care for the latter diagnosis. That information is available at the Center for Medicare and Medicaid Services (CMS) website. Another guide is to review the *American Journal of Medicine* article referred to in endnote 4 of this chapter for the section on "Geriatric Failure to Thrive." A third approach is to directly ask your physician: "How do I determine if I am dying of old age?" A specialist with a procedure to offer is likely to deflect this question. Your primary care doctor might hedge it. But a consultation with a geriatrician or a palliative care specialist, scheduled specifically for the purposes of discussing a prognosis, should help to address it.

With education and consultation you can foresee when some combination of poor performance status, advanced age, declining nutrition, comorbid illness, organ dysfunction, and repeat hospitalizations heralds that the end is approaching. This is the point when aggressive treatment is a zero-sum game: every day gained by treatment is actually lost, because it is spent in the hospital ICU when it could have been spent at home with family.

When you (patient, proxy, or family member) understand these principles, you can work backward to where you are on the performance scale and choose the course you want to take, toward medicalization or palliation.

MY FATHER'S FAILURE TO THRIVE

I had written Dad off immediately after our mother's death; I assumed he would go into an emotional decline, then a physical decline, and die of a broken heart within a year—but this was not the case. He did have an emotional decline, but then he rebounded. In fact, he had three excellent years before his aortic aneurysm repair and then three more good years following his aneurysm repair. The next two years, just before his death, were characterized by an accelerated decline and progressive debility.

Parsing, yet again, Sir William Osler's well-known quotation— "Pneumonia may well be called the friend of the aged. Taken off by it in an acute, short, not often painful illness, the old man escapes those 'cold gradations of decay' so distressing to himself and his friends."— helped me rationalize my despair when observing his deterioration during that phase. The second half of that quote highlights the grief felt by those observing dependence creep into and eventually take over the life of a proud man or woman. The first half of the quote reminds me of one exit opportunity that never came to pass for my father.

About one year before my father died, the physical limitations of his fatigue constricted the boundaries of his life to the confines of his apartment. With the exception of a rare restaurant meal (lunch only, as he could no longer sit for ninety minutes in the evening for a restaurant dinner), his once per month jazz evening, and the occasional opera broadcast, he was effectively homebound.

As a physician, I observed, analyzed, and integrated the clinical importance of his reduced circumstances. His social life was reduced to visits from family, relatives, and the occasional drop-in visitor. Although his appetite was excellent, his weight had leveled off at ten to twenty pounds below his maximum at the time of Mom's death. In terms of activities of daily living, he could not cook, clean, walk the length of a room, or bathe himself alone. He could barely toilet himself. At night, he used a bedside commode. During the day, he called for help to transfer to the bathroom commode. He could use a walker for a few yards, but generally relied on his caregivers to transfer him to a rolling chair to get from his bed to the table or elsewhere in the apartment. He could balance his checkbook and monitor his finances, but he needed help writing his checks and correspondence. He dictated his thoughts to his household help and signed the notes and checks with a "decrepit" (his lawyerly word) signature.

As a son, watching his decline distressed me greatly. As a physician, I did not need to review Medicare's eligibility requirements for hospice admission. I knew he was grieving his physical losses and struggling with the options to avoid prolonging his life and maybe to hasten his death. My siblings and I were willing to support this process as soon as he was ready to undertake it.

Dad had already discontinued routine visits with his primary care physician, and he eventually chose to discontinue visits with his oncologist as well as the monitoring of his abdominal aortic aneurysm. He was choosing to be aggressively passive. We understood and accepted that. He telephoned all his physicians independently, thanked them for their care, and said goodbye.

Eight months before his death, we were able to articulate that the end was coming even though precisely when was not yet in sight. Time was passing very slowly for us as he deteriorated and as my older sister negotiated more domestic assistance and home health care. Then, in a single week, he slipped twice and fell once while negotiating his way to the commode chair. It became clear to everyone that he needed help at night. And it was clear to me that the final decline had begun. "Old age" had become his terminal condition.

VISUALIZE THE QUALITY OF YOUR FINAL DAYS

While it is sufficiently easy to find what defines a median survival of six months for most conditions, it is emotionally and intellectually difficult to project that onto one's personal situation. However, it is well worth the effort—only those people who recognize their decline have the opportunity to take some control back from their treating physicians.

A chronic decline offers more time for this recognition to take place. Patients with a specific diagnosis, especially one that is universally recognized as a terminal illness (advanced cancer or end-stage heart disease, for example) have an advantage over those suffering the cumulative insults of old age. The former patients can easily get their hospice and home care team in place and trained for the inevitable. The latter have to do some extra work to get admitted to hospice. I will go through this process in detail in chapter 11: Hospice Care.

Practically speaking, it is a useful construct to divide terminally ill patients into three broad categories: those transitioning from a terminal diagnosis to a terminal condition with recognizable and quantifiable diseases (cancer, CHF, COPD, etc.); the sentient elderly who are failing to thrive (like my father); and the otherwise healthy but demented.

Recognizing the development of a terminal condition is critical because by doing so a patient can predict an exit opportunity and designate an exit strategy—an acute illness that, when ignored while superimposed on a terminal condition, will lead to a comfortable and timely passage.

Unfortunately, whenever these discussion points come up at a dinner conversation, some offended listener, usually a well-meaning friend or relative, argues, "You're just telling people to give up and die!" But that is not what I'm saying. What I am saying is, "Get educated; be aware; question aggressive therapeutic recommendations; question overly optimistic promises; exercise judgment." When the time is right for you, exercise aggressive passivity.

Harsh treatments toward the end of life might help a few patients live a little longer, but these same treatments have no effect (except side effects) for most elderly people, and they kill many people sooner than the disease itself. In fact, studies show that stage IV lung cancer patients live longer on average when they seek early palliative care than clinically matched patients seeking aggressive treatment.[6] Similar studies have been done in advanced breast cancer and pancreatic cancer patients with similar results. In those cases, choosing treatment over palliation increases the risk of painful and ineffective treatment, loss of control, and even an earlier death.

If you know your days are numbered, you know the "why" of your death. Ask yourself how you want to spend those days and visualize the "where" of your death. Do you want to spend them in a doctor's office, treatment center, nursing home, or hospital? Or would you prefer to spend those days with friends and family? Acknowledging a terminal diagnosis prepares a patient and their family to recognize a terminal condition. This is a variation on having a vision of how to die. At that point in the course of the illness at which further treatment might be counterproductive or side effects are intolerable, a person can exercise passivity, thereby influencing the "when" of death.

When an oncologist offers a treatment to "buy some time," consider ignoring that advice. Early hospice care buys more quality time, at home, with family and friends.

Accepting the inevitable is not giving up or giving in. It is taking action.

Things to Remember/Things to Consider

- Recognizing the reality of a disease is empowering.
- Communicating your vision unburdens your family.
- The recognition of a terminal diagnosis does not immediately consign you to a terminal condition.
- Know the "why" of your disease so that you can visualize the "where" and consider the "when" of its terminal evolution.
- Remember your option to limit or decline treatment.

Part Three

PRACTICAL ASPECTS OF
PLANNING FOR DEATH

Chapter Nine

The Value of Your Prognosis

In our rush not to abandon patients therapeutically at the end of life, we abandon them prognostically.

—Nicholas Christakis, MD

DOCTORS CRAVE MAKING diagnoses. With a diagnosis in hand they can develop a treatment plan. For the purposes of aggressive medical therapy, an accurate diagnosis is essential. But a diagnosis and treatment plan come with a prognosis—a forecast of the likely outcome of that diagnosis and plan—whether we want to recognize it or not. One of the purposes of this book is to encourage that a prognosis be recognized and discussed.

Earlier chapters in this book discuss the arc of disease, the transition from a terminal diagnosis to a terminal condition, and various deathbed scenarios. In a broad sense, the goal of those chapters was to inform the reader of what the future of a given disease might hold. It was to educate readers about the comparatively few chronic illnesses that cause death. It was to recognize when those illnesses transitioned from manageable to terminal. It was to outline the commonalities of the deathbed.

FROM GENERALITIES TO SPECIFICS

This chapter is designed to bring the generalities down to the specifics of a given individual. It is to help the reader to form a judgment about what is likely to happen in their future, given their illness and their particular circumstances. That is the definition of prognosis. If you know what is likely to happen then you can anticipate problems, make plans, and make contingency plans.

People make plans every day based on various sources of information—weather reports, train schedules, tide charts, stock indexes, and traffic patterns, to name a few. These are examples of information resources that use variable amounts of hard data, soft data, and speculation to help people anticipate, indeed to prognosticate, while they plan their day. However, there is much less attention paid by the average patient to all the information available to them about their illness and prognosis than there is to their diagnosis and to a blind faith in their doctor's recommendations. That is because, as patients with a recently diagnosed disease, we want to focus on the positive aspects of treatment after having been forced to accept the negative reality of the diagnosis.

PROGNOSIS: EITHER/OR OR ALONG A TIME LINE

The default position in American medicine is to diagnose and treat. For most medical illnesses the treatment is undertaken with the expectation of cure and long-term survival. For patients above a certain age or suffering from an advanced illness, that expectation might not be realistic and should be readjusted.

There are three variations of the concept of prognosis that tend to be conflated and should be teased apart for the benefit of the chronically ill. First, there is the prognostic concept of the manageability of their chronic disease. "What is the best I can expect from this new treatment of my chronic heart failure?" for example. Second, there is the prognostic concept of the curability of an acute illness superimposed on that chronic disease. "Can I expect to recover from this new blood clot in my lungs?" for example. Finally, there is the prognostic question, "How much time do I have left?"

The first concept was discussed in the preceding chapters. It has an either/or quality of adding a treatment or declining a treatment and analyzing the consequences. The second type of prognostication will be discussed shortly. It also has an either/or formulation. The third formulation is less about a treatment option and more about a time line. It is about life coming to a close and trying to predict when. Will it be sooner or later? It is sure to happen, but when? That will be discussed later in this chapter.

For the moment, let me tease apart these separate uses of the term "prognosis" with respect to my mother's diagnoses of frailty, pneumonia, and lung cancer. Her frailty was the initial chronic condition (as discussed in chapter 6) with which my parents coped but did not explore as a disease. Either we accepted the frailty or we fought it with a program of physical exercise and nutrition. Her pneumonia was an acute illness caused by, yet superimposed on, her lung cancer that, prognostically speaking, was likely to be cured by antibiotics. When her lung cancer was staged and determined to be advanced and incurable, she was immediately placed in the prognostic category of "how much time do I have left?" This is what I characterize as a single time line prognosis, an issue of median survival.

When I first met my parents after that diagnosis was established, they understood it was serious, but they had ignored or declined an in-depth discussion of that time line. When my mother was over the acute pneumonia, it was left to me to discuss her frailty, cancer, and life expectancy. Did I have the strength to be frank? How would I phrase it? Would I simply advise them that the median survival was ten months, or would I add that survival at one year was 20 percent? Does it soften the blow to rephrase it as half the people with your disease are dead in ten months and eight out of ten are dead in twelve months? Or should I emphasize that her overall weakness probably predicted a shorter overall life expectancy?

PROGNOSIS WHEN RECOVERY IS POSSIBLE

In my own practice, I used prognostic information to influence behavior on a frequent basis. Alcoholic liver disease is one of the best examples, because the treatment is abstinence and apart from the problems of withdrawal, there are no negative side effects of alcohol avoidance. Therefore, the risk–benefit analysis is particularly straightforward.

When a patient came to me for alcohol-induced liver disease,[1] I could plug their numbers into an algorithm and state, "If you stop drinking now, your lab tests will be normal in three months and your liver will regenerate by nine months; if you continue to drink, you are likely to die of liver failure in twelve months." That is a simple prognostication: a good prognosis if the patient chooses abstinence and a bad prognosis if they decline treatment. It is an either/or proposition.

Patients with other curable illnesses are willing to discuss treatment alternatives and variable prognoses. They want to know that if they choose treatment A, they can expect outcome B, or, if they choose treatment C, they can expect outcome D. In the case of alcoholic liver disease, the doctor has a diagnosis and the patient has a choice. There are, in fact, two prognoses. There is a good prognosis if the patient stops drinking and a bad prognosis if they do not. This dichotomy holds true of any reversible illness. For example, if a patient has appendicitis, they have a good prognosis if they agree to surgery and a bad prognosis if they do not.

PROGNOSIS WHEN RECOVERY IS NOT POSSIBLE

Alternatively, end-of-life circumstances focus on a single time line prognosis. That starts with the median survival for a given diagnosis and then comes into sharper focus as time passes and problems accumulate. Because complete recovery is not possible, decisions are reduced to either choosing treatment to "buy some time" or declining treatment to avoid side effects. The former comes with the potential for a longer life but the guaranteed discomforts of treatment and the risk of complication. The latter accepts the status quo and the presumption of more comfort.

When an elderly patient has a terminal illness, an advanced chronic illness, or frailty, there is only one outcome to anticipate. The prognosis is one of progressive decline. The time line might vary with different treatments, but the endpoint remains the same. More important, although progressive decline is guaranteed, the speed with which it occurs is not sure to be slowed by treatment. Complications of treatment might speed up the decline, rendering those treatments counterproductive.

Think about the brave woman I described in chapter 8. She was the woman with stage IV pancreatic cancer who asked and received prognostic information about her disease, treatment, and life expectancy. Advised that she had three to six months without chemotherapy and three to six additional months with chemotherapy, she declined treatment. She calculated that the additional time would be compromised by lower quality existence and she chose not to go there.

WITHHOLDING INFORMATION

It may seem harsh to some to put such numbers out in the open. Some physicians are tempted to withhold it. But knowledge is power, and sharing it is an act of common sense and occasionally of kindness. Yes, some patients do not want facts, but most are more comfortable with the information than without it. Some patients want to live in a state of denial, but they are the minority. In the absence of prognostic information most patients are anxious and uncomfortable as their minds ruminate over what is to come, and the minority of patients who seem more comfortable with denial are more likely to be subjected to futile treatment. In the presence of prognostic information, most patients appreciate the opportunity to work with the data to organize their remaining time.

Going back to my mother's diagnoses, I had uncomfortable choices to make. I have always felt that withholding a prognosis is as unethical as withholding a diagnosis.[2]

Excessively soft-pedaling a prognosis is a variation on withholding it. I reviewed her clinical parameters. I chose the hard-nosed construction of her prognosis and told her, "Fifty percent of patients with your disease will be dead in ten months and eighty percent will be dead in a year." I tried not to choke on the words, but I felt compelled to inform her. On the other hand, I did not emphasize that, based on her general weakness, she was less likely to get to ten months than a younger, fitter patient. That would have been too much.

I have not forgotten the soft sadness that moved across her face. "Am I dying, Sam?" Yes, I thought.

I shared her grief. It was clear that she had finally absorbed the enormity of my message. She had enough information to make educated decisions. She instinctively became passive about further medical treatment.

LESSONS FROM THE OLD WORLD VERSUS THE NEW WORLD

In my former practice in Washington, DC, I had the opportunity to consult with and treat people from all over the world. Frequently, successful immigrants or employees of foreign embassies brought their parents to the United States for treatment. This made for the interesting juxtaposition of two different perspectives and expectations, the Old World versus the New World. In such a setting it was common to be sitting with two generations, reviewing medical records from abroad, and discussing a malignant diagnosis. Frequently, the spokesman for the younger generation would ask me to follow the practices of the Old World physicians and withhold the actual diagnosis from the patient because they were too weak or sensitive to hear it right now. Usually this scenario occurred in the setting of a close-knit, protective, and well-intentioned family where the patient was living in a multigenerational household. Pathological denial was not a factor.

In this setting it was clear that the younger generation was trying to spare their parent, aunt, or uncle the shock of a serious diagnosis that would be perceived as a death sentence based on their Old World understanding of cancer or another serious illness. I presume they were struggling with the disconnect between their historical expectations and American expectations. Here we are bombarded with the hype surrounding the promise of American medical care. The presumption of the younger generation was that the patient could not handle the bad news nor take appropriate comfort in the good news offered by the promise of the American therapies.

This was not my experience. The Old World patients were much tougher than expected, having lived through more trials than their Americanized counterparts.

They seemed to know that much was outside their control, including serious illness. They were pleased to see what American medicine had to offer, but they were not blinded by overexpectations. They took their diagnoses well.

I always refused to withhold a diagnosis, and I never regretted it. Discussing the prognosis, a more nebulous subject, is more complicated and nuanced. In the end, however, a similarly direct approach was usually the best.

As noted elsewhere in this book, applying prognostic statistics about a population of patients to definitively predict the future of an individual patient is impossible. Physicians cannot plot the coordinates of our clinical perceptions or our patients' expectations. Patients cannot will where they will land on a survival curve.

To ignore statistics, however, is to deny the benefit of decades of research and observations. To ignore your prognosis is to deny the inevitable, and by fighting the inevitable, you guarantee overtreatment, futile therapies, and the loss of independence.

END-OF-LIFE PROGNOSIS

It is easier to predict the likelihood of a cure than to predict the duration of an illness. At the end of life, what is being predicted is the opposite of a cure; it is the length of time until treatment ultimately fails. It is the time of survival. The numbers expressed in the median survival are how many will be alive or dead in a given time frame, but they do not predict who will be alive or dead, nor does that single figure offer insight into the quality of life for survivors. As disease progresses and the time frame shortens, the accuracy of the forecast should improve, but it remains remarkably inexact. In one study of terminally ill patients being admitted to hospice care, only 20 percent of physicians' estimates of survival were correct. Seventeen percent were overly pessimistic (meaning patients lived longer than expected) and 63 percent were overly optimistic (meaning patients' lives were shorter than predicted—frequently by a factor of five).[3]

The fact that physicians are "systematically" optimistic when making end-of-life prognoses should contribute to your thinking. First, it might delay your consideration of hospice care. Second, it might inspire more ineffective, aggressive treatment. In the same study, experienced, specialized physicians who did not have a long-term relationship with the patient offered the most accurate predictions. Therefore, when concerned with a recommendation for aggressive treatment, consider a prognostic reality check with a second opinion from a disinterested party. I served this role in the stomach cancer patient described in chapter 8.

One of the best examples of prognostic information used well occurred late in my career when I had the opportunity to consult on the care of an acquaintance in Washington. The patient was a seventy-five-year-old woman who had received most of her care elsewhere. Her first visit occurred one January when she came to see me for vague abdominal pain, appetite loss, and unusual fatigue after hosting her family for the holidays. She was an elegant, reserved woman, but without pretensions. I learned little of medical value from taking her history.

I learned a lot during the physical examination, however. The moment I touched her liver (which was rock hard and lumpy) I knew that she had terminal cancer. Whether it was a primary liver cancer or a metastatic cancer from the lungs, breasts, pancreas, or elsewhere was of marginal importance relative to her life expectancy. What was important was that this disease would now define her existence. She could read that on my face.

When further tests and a biopsy revealed widespread bile duct cancer (metastatic bile duct cancer—cholangiocarcinoma—has a prognosis similar to advanced pancreatic cancer), she and her husband had a particularly frank discussion with me. Most important to her prognosis, the CAT scan showed pockets of thick fluid and deposits of cancer in her abdomen, surrounding her bowel and forecasting multiple future episodes of bowel obstruction, a particularly painful and unpleasant situation at the end of life.

She interviewed several oncologists and planned to try chemotherapy to "buy some time." Unfortunately, in the middle of the night following her first chemo treatment she awoke with an attack of nausea. She sat up in bed, clutched her chest, exhaled audibly, and expired. Most spouses would have panicked and called 911, even though there was nothing that could be done. Her husband, recognizing a fatal event in a terminally ill patient, wisely called her physicians for instructions, thereby sparing her the futility of attempted CPR and the indignity of an ambulance ride to the nearest emergency room to be pronounced dead by the ER physician.[4]

My guess was that she died instantaneously of a pulmonary embolus.

The compassionate communication of the prognosis in terms of short life expectancy and poor quality of life allowed this couple to benefit by an "exit opportunity" that was uncomplicated by futile emergency attention.

MY FATHER: USING PROGNOSTIC INFORMATION TO HIS ADVANTAGE

When my father was eighty-three, his oncologist ordered a CAT scan to monitor his indolent lymphoma. Incidentally, his abdominal aortic aneurysm (AAA), a ballooned blood vessel at risk for rupture, was noticed for the first time. Standard care is to set up a program to monitor the size and rate of growth of such an aneurysm with the goal of surgical repair when the risk of rupture exceeds the risk of surgery.

Two years after my mother's death, my father was eighty-eight and still living independently. Routine studies now showed the aneurysm had expanded and repair must be considered. His primary physician set him up with two surgical consultations.

I introduced him to an online information service, UpToDate.[5]

At his advanced age, definitive surgical repair carried a high risk. Although he was still comparatively vigorous, the risk of a complication was high and the probability of a setback was even higher. A large abdominal surgery, even if performed flawlessly, would require days in the ICU and possibly weeks in a hospital or nursing home. This, in turn, would result in weakness from which he was not likely to fully recover.

Endovascular aneurysm repair (EVAR) was a lower risk alternative, however. This was like a cardiac catheterization and stent insertion but on a larger-scale blood vessel. It is a procedure that can be done on an outpatient basis, and it dramatically reduces the risk of a rupture for five years or more, the idea being that during that time another medical issue would develop and carry him away.

But did he want to be treated at all? Decades before, he had seen a legal client die of an aneurysm. He knew that most people died fairly quickly and he wondered about the wisdom of leaving his aneurysm untreated.

"If you want to die of an aneurysm, here is how the rupture will play out," I said. I went on to describe my perceptions of the process in significant detail.

"The facts are that it is not such a bad plan. Fifty percent of patients will die before getting to the hospital. The pain will be severe but brief. If you get to the hospital you will be medicated with morphine. An additional fifteen to twenty-five percent will die before surgery is possible. Assuming you decline surgery, death is certain, but for about one quarter of those who have survived long enough to decline surgery, death can take up to four days."

Two points resonated with my father. The death scenario was

usually quick and, by declining surgery, it was certain. The pain could be managed with morphine.

"So why would I want to fix this?"

"Dad, your granddaughter is pregnant. If you want to increase the chances of holding your first great-grandchild, you should get it repaired."

Ultimately that argument held sway. He had it repaired with the stent procedure. Six months later he traveled to Connecticut to visit his great-granddaughter. The power of prognostic information helped him make the decision. Five years later, another CAT scan to follow up his lymphoma showed the repair breaking down and the aorta expanding. His doctors recommended a repeat procedure, although how long it would be beneficial was less clear than with the initial repair. This time Dad took the updated information, thanked his doctors, and declined further intervention.

RESEARCHING YOUR PROGNOSIS

Your physicians are the most important resource that you have for understanding your prognosis. But it is the rare physician that will push this information at you. Only a minority will discuss it willingly. Part of that hesitation is because long discussions are not well compensated. Another part is the patronizing perspective that patients cannot really absorb the information. If pushed, most physicians will acquiesce. If they don't, consider another physician. It is your right to be informed. Don't take no for an answer.

In addition to your medical consultants, you should know that online resources have been growing in number and in reliability. During my career, as the Internet grew, I routinely advised my patients to avoid surfing the web. There was too much unregulated misinformation that could obscure facts and confuse decision making. Over the years, however, many reliable sites have been established. UpToDate is just one example. Your doctor can steer you to others.

More important, disease specific sites that are affiliated with responsible treatment centers (Memorial Sloan-Kettering Cancer Center, for example) offer diagnosis specific prognosis algorithms.[6] For example, a patient with pancreatic cancer can go to such a site, as recommended by their consulting physician, type in their diagnosis and their clinical parameters (height, weight, age, comorbid illnesses, tobacco use, metastases, etc.), and get a prognosis independent of their doctor's opinion. I recommend the use of such sites, not to replace a discussion with your physician or family member, but to amplify it with objective information that can be a starting point for a more personalized perspective.

Because this book focuses on "old age" as a disease and a potentially terminal condition, I recommend another site: ePrognosis.ucsf.edu.org. Associated with the University of California in San Francisco Medical School, it offers a tool for elderly patients to use in several ways.[7]

Most important, it offers an algorithm for elderly patients without a specific diagnosis to estimate the probability of surviving for a given period of time. After entering similar demographic, physical, and comorbidity details the patient gets a graph-like representation of how many people in an equally matched cohort will be alive in a given time frame. If you, or your doctor, choose a six- to twelve-month time frame it might be used for hospice eligibility.

For example, if you learn that 75 percent of a matched group passes away by the twelve-month mark, then it is likely that a hospice application is appropriate.

Finally, when dealing with an advanced chronic illness or frailty, reviewing the government guidelines that qualify a patient for the financial benefits of hospice care can be very informative. These are known as the Local Coverage Determinants (LCDs). From a prognostic perspective, the condition described in the LCDs for each of the chronic diseases establishes the government's assessment of a median survival of six months.[8]

CLOSING THOUGHTS ON PROGNOSIS

At the beginning of this chapter, I emphasized the importance of diagnosis and prognosis as pillars of medical care, especially aggressive care where the intent to treat for a cure is being practiced. An accurate diagnosis leads to a treatment plan, and that combination establishes a prognosis.

With the guidance of your physician, that information is of enormous value. Although the statistics, charts, graphs, or figures do not predict what will happen to any given patient, I want to pass on what my college chemistry professor emphasized when discussing entropy: "On average, the most likely thing will happen." You should educate yourself about what is likely, discuss the particulars with your physician, and plan accordingly. Then you can relish the better than expected outcomes and accept the less favorable outcomes.

Things to Remember/Things to Consider

- You have a prognosis whether you choose to recognize it or not.
- Ignoring your prognosis encourages denial, promotes the momentum to treat, and often results in futile and painful therapies.
- Discuss your prognosis with your physician.
- If your physician declines to discuss it, ask for a referral to a geriatrician or palliative care physician who will talk with you.

Chapter Ten

The Hard Conversation

I believe it is crucial to be forthright and honest with my patients and their families. Too many of my colleagues have mastered the art of verbal subterfuge and obfuscation for fear of squelching hope or in order to avoid difficult discussions, but withholding information from patients and their families prevents them from making informed decisions.

—Angelo Volandes, MD

E ND-OF-LIFE WISHES CAN be as specific as refusing mechanical ventilation, as broad as "I want you to do everything to keep me alive as long as I can read and enjoy the front page of the newspaper," or as nebulous as my father's express desire to avoid nursing home placement. But in order for these wishes to have meaning and to take on substance, they must be communicated to the family and, where they are separate, the agent. Books, journals, and films have come to popularly refer to that communication as "The Conversation" (Angelo Volandes) or "The Hard Conversation" (Atul Gawande). I use both terms, depending on how late in the course of an illness the conversation takes place. The longer the delay in starting and the less frequent the conversations are, overall, the harder they become.

It is always difficult to discuss disease, dying, and death, because the issue of facing reality is routinely intertwined with dashing "hope." But having The Conversation doesn't have to be hard and, later in the course of the illness, having The Hard Conversation should not be impossible. This chapter will try to unravel this process.

HOW TO START

Before a serious illness occurs, The Conversation is always hypothetical. Once one is staring illness in the face, The Conversation can be harder to begin because now the possibility of a crisis looms. But to avoid having it is to cede control to others and to hide from reality. Alternatively, to pursue it is to assert some control. By opening The Conversation, one is expressing care and concern for all parties involved in the decision making. If the family pursues it, they are showing that they care for the patient and want to protect them from unwanted or ineffective treatment. If the patient pursues it they are demonstrating care for their family by sharing their vision and decreasing the burden of future decision making.

There are many ways to open The Conversation. The easiest and most common is to segue from a practical discussion of a health-related matter to a deeper discussion of end-of-life goals, but other starting points include a legal perspective, a medical perspective, and finally a moral perspective. Some form of denial is always a factor in postponing the process, but it should never be delayed to "protect" the patient. Usually, the discussion gets delayed because it is easier to ignore problems than to engage them. When in doubt, one must blunder ahead, taking care to be respectful and trying to avoid a brow-beatingly specific agenda.

MY FATHER AND THE FIRST CONVERSATION

My father did not shrink from The Conversation. He did not, however, embrace it. He always approached it tangentially. We usually started it by discussing a practical problem.

With the exception of redrafting his advance directive, about twelve years prior to his death, the first Hard Conversation that was focused on my father occurred six years later and revolved around the subject of a call button. At the time, he was living alone in a single-story apartment in a residential hotel. At eighty-seven years of age, he was not yet physically frail, but he was a real fall risk. He was taking three prescription medications (for blood pressure, anxiety, and pain) that were associated with an increased incidence of falls, and he was suffering from a peripheral neuropathy (nerve damage in the legs).[1]

We had frequently danced around the subject of safety in the apartment, especially in the kitchen and the shower. We had fitted his shower with extra handgrips, nonskid floor strips, and a waterproof chair. Then it happened, the fall I mentioned in chapter 3.

He cracked his head on the kitchen floor but broke nothing and did not lose consciousness. The result was a conversation themed around the acquisition of a safety call button, something that in principle he did not want, because at the time he was still able to get himself up from the floor after such a fall, and absent a major injury. By moving the subject from a fall and a call button to the practical reality of dealing with a fall with injury, it became part of The Conversation.

Should he be unable to get himself up, my father was adamant that he would prefer to die a painless death on the floor of his kitchen rather than call for help. I offered to describe the pathophysiology of death following an unattended household fall. I explained to him that assuming the fall resulted in painless unconsciousness, the altered mental status would be perpetuated by renal failure and death would result. My father was hopeful.

Unfortunately, his assumption of painless unconsciousness was a false hope. I explained that a painful fracture was a realistic possibility and death could be a long time coming.

A second outcome, more likely than painless loss of consciousness, would be a fall without injury, but at a time when he was unable to raise himself from the floor to a bed or chair. This is a significant social and physical development that ultimately affects everyone lucky enough to reach an advanced age. The sense of helplessness it engenders should be a warning sign to a patient trying to live independently. It is a negative milestone. Left alone for too long, that person will die slowly of dehydration. More likely, a caretaker, friend, or family member will find them but only after many unhappy hours or days. To be unable to independently rise from the floor to a standing position is part of my definition of frailty, and its recognition is a takeoff point for The Hard Conversation.

Dad temporarily continued his resistance to a safety alert button, preferring to experiment with a daily morning call with a neighbor. But over time this proved more cumbersome and challenging than expected. Ultimately, the dream of toughing it out on the floor of his kitchen faded, and he acquired the button. By then he had verbalized many of his end-of-life hopes.

Early in his widower status, Dad was a tough talker about "waking up dead" and avoiding hospitalization or nursing home convalescence. To make that point, he began wearing Mom's former DNR bracelet. We revisited the "waking up dead" theme many times and in many forms. To die in one's sleep is considered very desirable by those elderly who are emotionally prepared for death in general. The assumption is that it is painless and quick. Few give thought to the potential for seizures, aspiration, and choking that might be the actual modus exodus during the night in question or, for that matter, following a "suicide pill." Fewer still give thought to how comparatively rare this outcome is among the old but not yet disabled or debilitated.

My conversations with my sisters on this subject emphasized the agreement we shared to delay a 911 call should he be found unresponsive, but comfortable, some morning. "Do not call 911 until he is cold and blue" was our mantra. In conversations with Dad, I emphasized the unlikely possibility of prematurely dying in his sleep and his need for another plan.

The thrust of these paragraphs is to point out that several things that commonly occur in old age are often underappreciated as signs of decline but merit further consideration. When a family has to hire household help to protect their loved one, when an elderly person is unable to pick themselves up from a fall, when a safety call button is considered, and when the "waking up dead" desire is expressed, it's tempting to dismiss them as mundane developments. These are not mundane. They are in fact important developments and ideal opportunities to seize for beginning The Conversation.

TIME LINE FOR THE CONVERSATION

Whenever it takes place, The Conversation changes along a predictable time line. As time passes and disease progresses, The Conversation becomes more complicated and more detailed. Early in life it is a hypothetical issue and is framed by the creation of a simple advance directive in young adulthood. Later in life it's revisited at the time of a medical issue or hospitalization. Finally, late in life, it becomes The Hard Conversation with the realization that the specter of death looms large.

Though the difficulties associated with The Hard Conversation increase with the proximity to death, the more frequently the discussions occur throughout life, the easier they are, in general. The later the discussions occur in the trajectory of an illness, the harder they are to initiate because they are now intertwined with the actuality of death and the end of hope. But the closer to death these discussions occur, and the more frequently they are reviewed and revised, the more power and influence they have to assert your control over the process of moving toward a more peaceful death.

THE LEGAL PERSPECTIVE

One way to start The Conversation is to approach it as an addendum to another legal issue, such as the creation or revision of a last will and testament. This usually occurs at the time of a marriage or the incorporation of a business, when a lawyer's advice is being sought for non-health-related matters. At this time, a good lawyer will help create a will and an advance directive at the same time, generally by supplying a simple form that can be easily filled out with a few responses and the quick, almost reflexive checking of boxes.

The advantage of starting here is that the boilerplate offered is likely to be consistent with the jurisdictional standards. It is likely to consist of choices about what to do in the event of a terminal illness in conjunction with an inability to communicate (coma or brain damage), including checkboxes for things like CPR, mechanical ventilation, artificial nutritional support, dialysis, and the like. The document also allows for the identification of an agent who will act as a durable power of attorney. At this point, these questions and answers are hypothetical and they are comparatively easy. This is not The Hard Conversation. But it is a start, and it is a step that should be taken.

THE MEDICAL PERSPECTIVE

From the medical perspective, the most common way to back into an advance directive is to be hospitalized for an elective surgery or medical treatment. Courtesy of the Patient Self-Determination Act of 1991, federal law requires hospitals to provide information about advance health care directives but does not require that a patient make any choices. It also states that patients without advance directives cannot be discriminated against. Based on the rules and regulations of the hospital or medical staff, it falls to the admitting physician to discuss specific decisions. Most hospitals, at a minimum, require that the admitting physician obtain a "yes or no" decision about cardiopulmonary resuscitation and record the choice on the chart. This is not The Hard Conversation, but if you are aware of this requirement you can use it as a starting point. Unfortunately, because this rule does not have the force of law behind it, many physicians ignore or delay the discussion. Because, in the absence of a written order, the hospital's default position is full cardiopulmonary resuscitation, the result is that many patients are exposed to potential CPR despite advanced age or advanced illness.

The best time to start the medical discussion is before a hospitalization, and the best practice is to involve a trusted physician. The proactive patient might call their physician and ask to review their advance directive with a more focused and detailed discussion in mind. If the patient is passive and the family is concerned, most physicians will start that conversation at the family's request. These requests move you closer to the actual Hard Conversation. Prior to October 2015, these conversations with physicians were not compensated, so many physicians had not felt encouraged to pursue them.

If there is no primary care physician (PCP) to lean on, or if the

PCP is reluctant to help, seek out a consultation with a geriatrician. It should be part of a geriatrician's professional practice to address end-of-life issues. A geriatrician should be well versed in starting and pursuing conversations about end of life long before the average physician is comfortable doing so. A patient or family member can drive this agenda, and coming prepared will facilitate the process.

The Stanford Letter Project (SLP) is an outgrowth of the Palliative Care Department at the Stanford University School of Medicine.[2] It supplies a template for a letter from a patient to their physician outlining common end-of-life choices. The PDF can be downloaded in several languages. It is not a legal document, but it is a good icebreaker. It will ease all parties into the process.

Another medical circumstance that leads directly to The Hard Conversation is one I alluded to in chapter 8, where I was asked to give a second opinion about a patient with stomach cancer. When a surgeon is consulted to operate on the inoperable or a specialist consultant is asked to treat the incurable, the new consultant can offer an unvarnished opinion, a new and objective perspective that introduces a dose of reality and jump-starts The Hard Conversation. Of course, in this situation, The Conversation has been delayed too long and some benefits of early decision making (e.g., early hospice admission, simplification of medications, avoidance of unnecessary treatments or doctor visits, etc.) will have been lost. But this opportunity should still be embraced to avoid further medicalization.

THE MORAL PERSPECTIVE

The moral responsibility as to when and how to have The Hard Conversation transcends even the most difficult clinical situations. The patient (or agent) and his or her doctor share this responsibility. Before a patient (or agent) can make an informed decision, they must have the necessary information. With respect to end-of-life decisions, it is the physician's moral responsibility to advise the patient (or agent)—within their limits of understanding—of the clinical situation and to seek answers to questions about therapy. It is the responsibility of the patient (or agent) to respond.

It might be legal and expedient to overtreat an uninformed patient who has not otherwise offered limiting guidelines, but it is morally wrong to do so. In the event of a patient's mental decline, it is immoral to allow the agent to be inadequately informed. It is unethical for them to avoid The Hard Conversation with the patient's medical team and other family members simply because it is an uncomfortable conversation.

Family members should understand that it is immoral to hide information from patients and thereby delay end-of-life directives. It is immoral to patronize, indulge, and "protect" the old and infirm, but sentient, from scientific fact.

The Hard Conversation occurs when reality is faced head-on. When a chronic disease is recognized, a terminal diagnosis is made, a proposed surgery or other treatment regimen has an unfavorable risk–benefit ratio, or when age and declining performance status require lifestyle adjustments, then The Hard Conversation is the moral, ethical, and practical course of action.

PERSONALITY DISORDERS AND INTRACTABLE DENIAL

When discussing end-of-life issues in terminal situations, some degree of denial is universal and natural. This denial is usually overcome with a little prodding. However, some patients and families cannot face reality, and in those cases, unfortunately, The Hard Conversation never occurs. The frequent result is a death characterized by excessive treatments involving prolonged life support with real pain and suffering but without real hope of benefit.

In my own practice, such perpetual denial was rare. Most of my patients chose to stay with me, or to pursue second opinions with me, because they appreciated a straightforward approach.

Physicians continued to send patients for consultation because they knew they would get realistic recommendations. I suspect that most patients who wanted pie-in-the-sky promises found their way to other physicians, but not all.

One problem patient, whom I will call Sarah, refused to listen to realistic recommendations. She didn't face her illnesses head-on until she had spent many weeks in an ICU. When she finally realized that death was upon her, she left behind many unhappy people and several frivolous lawsuits.

The story of Sarah began with her referral for iron deficiency anemia (a low blood count resulting from blood loss and inadequate iron intake) at the age of eighty. She came from a "concierge physician" who had been caring for her tobacco-induced chronic lung disease. Sarah also suffered from high blood pressure, heart disease, osteoporosis (weak bones), gallstones, and frailty. It was clear from the referral letter and telephone conversations that she was a difficult patient who didn't follow medical advice. She also had a complicated domestic situation, living with her unemployed son and his wife.

I recommended a colonoscopy to exclude colon cancer as the most common and serious cause of blood loss, followed by an endoscopy (a scope exam of the stomach) to look for an ulcer or the comparatively uncommon stomach cancer.[3] Sarah adamantly declined a colonoscopy, saying, "I would rather die of colon cancer than have that test," based on a rational but exaggerated fear of the preparation. Fortunately, her endoscopy revealed a benign ulcer, and this proved to be an adequate explanation for her anemia. She improved with iron supplements and stomach acid suppressants, and I became her hero for postponing the colonoscopy.

She started sending me progressively expensive presents of wine and cheese. This situation devolved to include inappropriate and exaggerated letters of appreciation. In return, she expected special treatment. Her son would accompany her on her office visits. They rarely agreed on anything, and they frequently argued.

Sarah declined routine follow-up endoscopies, and her ulcer waxed and waned as she took her medications unreliably. I returned all the gifts and retained her letters for potential proof of unbalanced behavior. Ultimately, because of her distortion of the doctor-patient relationship, including multiple unreasonable demands about who could treat her and when, I fired her as a patient.[4]

Ten to twelve months later, she was hospitalized for what proved to be the last of several "gallbladder attacks."[5] She had refused gallbladder surgery in the past based on semi-rational discussions with her son. The physicians accepted this decision because her lungs were so diseased that the surgical risk was very high. Fortunately for her, her previous episodes had improved with antibiotics. This time the attack did not improve. When evidence of gallbladder gangrene developed, the surgeon's hand was forced. Sarah and her son were presented with the choice to operate or to palliate with pain medications—the emergency surgery exit option. Having studiously avoided any discussions of mortality despite multiple ICU admissions over the preceding months, they chose surgery.

Sarah survived the difficult surgery and spent several more weeks in the ICU and on the hospital wards, but before being discharged she developed a recurrent pneumonia and returned to the ICU. After several days of aggressive treatment, she turned to her physicians and in a cogent moment without her son's concurrence she asked to be changed to a Do Not Resuscitate status. Having duly documented that in the chart, when her heart stopped a few days later, her physicians did not attempt to resuscitate her, despite her son's frantic remonstrations.

Her son was distraught, but not because his mother had suffered needlessly and predictably. They could have justified hospice care months before her death. Rather, he was distraught because their codependent relationship promoted denial and prevented them from addressing the inevitability of her death.

Sarah's story is an example of extreme, indeed pathologic, dysfunction. But it exemplifies how badly things can turn out without a realistic discussion of disease, prognosis and treatment plans.

A less dysfunctional and more common example is well documented in *Can't We Talk about Something More Pleasant?* by Roz Chast. In this illustrated book, Ms. Chast documents her parents' resistance to dealing with The Hard Conversation. Though they ultimately died non-medicalized deaths and end-of-life discussions would not have made their deaths "better," I suspect Ms. Chast would have felt better if she had had an understanding that her parents were grounded in reality and if she were confident a medicalized death and its attendant suffering was likely to be avoided.

An important lesson from her book, unstated but inferred, is that her gentle but persistent attempts to discuss end-of-life choices did not prompt a definitive conversation, although it might have nudged her parents toward slow medical decisions and away from aggressive treatments. Alternatively, browbeating patients is counterproductive because it shuts down communication. It is also morally inappropriate.

When I was an intern, a supervising physician dressed me down for over-aggressively recommending a course of treatment to an indigent patient. The elderly woman was declining blood thinner therapy in the face of phlebitis (blood clots in the legs) and a pulmonary embolus (blood clot in the lungs). It was unclear to me that she fully understood the consequences of her decision, and I wanted her to accept my recommendations. I would not take her "no thank you" for an answer.

Through that experience, I learned the hard way that people should be allowed to decline intervention if they have been informed of the risks and benefits of treatment and the consequences of inaction. This principle also applies to the give and take of The Hard Conversation. Doctors and agents cannot morally avoid introducing the end-of-life discussion, but patients can refuse to participate beyond their comfort zone. Doctors and agents must lead and educate, but they should not force the agenda or demand a certain conclusion.

Recently, a former patient told me the story of her father's death from congestive heart failure. He refused to discuss end-of-life issues with her because he felt trapped in caring for his agoraphobic wife. Ultimately, after multiple and cyclical hospitalizations and another impending ICU admission, the daughter gently prevailed on her father and the critical care physician to consult with a palliative care specialist. This rapidly and successfully evolved into a hospice care admission, and the daughter saved her father from further fruitless overtreatment. Her story shows how working around the margins of the problem can ultimately create the opportunity to influence the final decisions. One cannot mandate The Conversation, but one must continue to prod it along.

Without badgering anyone, by accepting that some initial degree of denial is normal, and by remaining sensitive to the patients' cultural, social, and educational backgrounds, it is the physician's job to assert that in our medical culture the patient, if competent, makes the decisions. To do so, the patient must be informed. The Hard Conversation has to happen in order for doctors to treat people ethically, morally, and responsibly. I can't remember an emotionally stable patient from any of the diverse backgrounds in my practice who was unwilling to handle the choices when they were finally informed.

STRATEGIES FOR CONVERSATIONS

Practically speaking, most grounded people are willing to discuss end-of-life issues within sensible limits. Most patients have already considered these issues somewhere in the recesses of their minds. I found that most newcomers to my practice (and all returning regulars) were quite prepared to have circumspect end-of-life conversations, despite "protective" family members. But many patients are resistant to detailed discussions, and family members and agents must be aware of the strategies for initiating and restarting them regularly.

Every death of a friend or acquaintance is an opportunity to broach the subjects of funeral and burial plans. Every domestic development, be it a fall, a fender-bender, a checkbook error, or a cooking disaster, is a reason to discuss long-term care plans. That can morph into a discussion of limits and limitations to such care. Every hospitalization of everyone you know, friend or relative, is an opportunity to update The Conversation. Remember, not every conversation must be codified in a written advance directive. Not every conversation has to close with a decision about cardiopulmonary resuscitation. A general discussion of what is too much treatment and what is too little treatment will slowly paint a picture that the family can share, and painting that picture in an atmosphere of trust and compassion will serve as a useful verbal directive to an agent that has the same power as a written directive.

Of course, the stress of an active illness for any given admission might absorb the energy needed for a detailed or nuanced exploration of the advance directive's clauses early in the course of a hospitalization, but during the recovery phase, when relief is in sight and the memories of hospitalization are fresh, such a discussion can be had. This is an ideal time to review the overall experience and discuss treatments to be avoided in the future, particularly because new and unsuspected information about a patient is often generated during elective and emergency admissions.

For example, a common scenario from my past would be the hospitalization for a hip fracture of a previously healthy seventy-year-old. Typically, the patient would arrive via the emergency room having left their advance directive at home. Depending on operating room availability, compounding health problems, and the surgeon's schedule, the patient would be expedited to the floor or directly to the OR. During these hectic hours, dozens of documents would be signed and witnessed without detailed review. One of these documents would be the hospital's boilerplate advance directive. Such a form offers an abbreviated checklist of options to consider "in the event of" cardiovascular collapse or coma. These options would include orders to perform CPR (or not) and choices for (or against) mechanical ventilation, feeding tubes, hemodialysis, and so on.

In the absence of a pre-existing advance directive, this checklist would be rapidly filled in, signed, and witnessed. The path of least resistance would be to check "yes" to CPR and move on. The patient and family then return to the details of the impending surgery and the more pressing matters of getting through the day. After surgery, previously underappreciated illnesses will need to be addressed.

For example, the "previously healthy" seventy-year-old is likely to be found to have underlying heart disease based on the anesthesiologist's evaluation, high blood pressure, an abnormal heart rhythm, or fluid accumulation during surgery. It is also possible that the underlying conditions that led to the fall and the fracture will have long-term implications. Cerebrovascular disease, diabetes, osteoporosis, and neurological disorders are common co-diagnoses that appear on the medical record after such an event. It's important to explore these as issues of concern in future iterations of the advance directive and not to ignore them.

If a patient suffers a complication of the surgery or hospitalization such as pneumonia, an ileus (paralyzed bowel), a hospital-acquired infection (HAI), a blood clot, or a bleeding episode, then prolonged rehabilitation might be needed.

Every hospitalization or nursing home stay supplies experiences that should be mined for a patient's perspective on their future care. Indeed, every death or illness of close friends or relatives should be similarly evaluated. Even if the details are unclear, speculation can be informative. "How many courses of chemotherapy did Aunt Sally have?" is a perfectly legitimate discussion point. "I heard that she was in lots of pain." "I heard that she was [or was not] nauseated." These are valuable starting points for personal reflection. Because they involve third parties, they are slightly less threatening, but they keep the conversation alive.

There exist multiple online resources for promoting end-of-life conversations. I mention several in the Resource List section.

HOPE AND THE HARD CONVERSATION

In the absence of pathological denial, resistance to the most difficult conversations, especially when facing serious illness late in life, is fundamentally about losing hope for an extended future.

Several years ago, an English friend was diagnosed with pancreatic cancer at the age of sixty-two. Upon diagnosis, he started a long course of chemotherapy and radiation therapy. Because we did not know how long he would live or what course his disease would take, we visited England ten months later. Fortunately, he was holding up quite well, and we subsequently traded visits every six to eight months for three years.

At the time of our last visit, he was still going to work every day, but his other activities were quite limited. Two weeks before our trip, he was hospitalized for gastrointestinal bleeding. When we arrived, he had just been informed that the blood loss from his bowels was the result of a malignant ulcer in his duodenum. The pancreatic cancer had burrowed into his intestines. My first thought was that of a physician: his terminal condition had arrived.

While our wives were off sharing their sorrow in another room, he and I chatted. From a distance, I overheard his wife say, "We cannot stop treatment; that would mean we have given up hope." I wanted to tell him what the recent developments meant to me. A malignant ulcer at this stage in his disease meant there was no further chance of long-term survival. More treatment would be futile. But I was his friend and not his doctor. I could not bring myself to say something that would deflate his courageous optimism. Furthermore, it was not my place to do so.

Based on those conversations, I was afraid he would be subjected to uncomfortable and ineffective therapy. Fortunately, the common sense of his British physicians, his stiff upper lip, and his wife's intelligence prevailed. Without clearly vocalizing a change of direction, they moved toward supportive care and then palliative care. He died in the hospital, in hospice care, three weeks after our visit, approximately three and a half years after his terminal diagnosis.

His cancer was premature, and I know that hope for a cure must not be stifled prematurely. But when his cancer changed from a terminal diagnosis to a terminal condition, it was critical that he and his family found the strength to move from a false hope to an acceptance of the inevitable, thus sparing him fruitless treatment and prolonged suffering.

In the health care setting, the automatic assumption is that hope exists solely for a positive outcome, at least long-term survival and at best a cure. The universal tendency among family members to admonish elderly patients to "not give up hope" must be tempered with reality. The seduction of "medical progress" and the fear of death delay The Hardest Conversation and blind us to the consequences of the false hope born of excessive treatment. Those consequences are the pain and suffering of ineffective care.

There is a temptation in the medical setting to pair the absence of hope for a cure with hopelessness. This represents an absoluteness that does not exist elsewhere. In a non-medical setting, we can see various degrees of hope. For example, we can hope to win the lottery and we can enjoy the anticipation following the purchase of such a ticket, but we understand that those riches are not likely to become our own. When hope for a longer life is no longer realistic, hope for other attributes of a good life and a good death (acceptance, appreciation, reconciliation, and forgiveness) become a potentially rewarding alternative.

A different way of avoiding hopelessness at the end of life was suggested to me by a friend while we were discussing the death of her close friend and neighbor, a woman with whom I informally consulted. That person had a "good death"—at home, in peace, and surrounded by friends and family. But death is always messy, and enduring the dying process is always hard. We were reviewing the trials of that death when my friend made reference to her own Buddhist practices, including meditation and "being in the moment." She suggested that the mindfulness of being in the moment was life without future, without desire, without anticipation, and, therefore, without the burden of hope, hopelessness, or denial. Certainly, "being in the moment" is emphasized to all seriously ill patients, and it becomes progressively important as death nears.

Whether spiritually or as a secularist, living in the moment acknowledges that time is no longer the objective. Living in the moment weakens the grip that hope plays in promoting denial and strengthens the role that life plays at its end.

We believe patients don't want to be reminded of their imminent death, and yet they are quietly thinking of it with regularity. Based on my experience with the premature death of my friend or the post-mature deaths of my parents, I acknowledge that The Hard Conversation is always difficult to initiate and frequently difficult to pursue. I have long tried to create a philosophical argument that breaks down any barrier to frank discussions about end-of-life issues, but " losing hope" and the fear of "hopelessness" always intervene. I am left only with the practical argument that the alternative—painful, futile treatment inspired by a fear of hopelessness—is worse. I swallow my anxiety and plunge forward.

THE CONVERSATION, CONTROL, AND A GOOD DEATH

When the attributes of "a good death" are analyzed, researchers conclude that the most important characteristic is some degree of "control."[6] The dying patient wants to assert some influence on this process. To do so, they need a vision and a plan. Although the moment of death is irreversible and, at that instant, uncontrollable, the days, weeks, months, and even years leading up to that moment can be managed for the aging patient to include more self-assertion and less overtreatment. Planning is essential for control, and The Conversation is essential for a plan.

How The Conversation begins, be it from a legal, medical, or practical springboard, is less important than the recognition of its moral imperative. How it is advanced is less critical than the fact that it is advanced at all. The Conversation shares a vision and this, in turn, inspires planning. Together, a vision and a plan replace denial with understanding, mitigate fear, convert hopelessness into control, and reduce the family's burden of responsibility. When The Conversation is advanced, unnecessary tests and treatments are avoided.

Things to Remember/Things to Consider

- Using your vision, blunder ahead starting The Conversation, gently but repetitively.
- Engage your physician in the process. Try the Stanford Letter Project.
- Start The Conversation with a discussion of someone else's medical problems, a home health care issue (such as the need for a safety call button), or the practical aspects of an end-of-life issue (such as the family gravesite), and morph that into a discussion about end-of-life wishes.
- Recognize denial.
- Consider formulations of hope beyond that of a longer life to include control, comfort, closure, and affirmation.

Chapter Eleven

Hospice Care

Every day is a fresh beginning,
Listen my soul to the glad refrain;
And spite of old sorrows and older sinning,
Troubles forecasted and possible pain;
Take heart with the day and begin again.

—Susan Coolidge
Adopted as an unofficial hospice poem

———————

T HE MOST WORTHWHILE medical treatments will improve the quality of life as well as the quantity. No test is acceptably safe if it does not have the specific effect of leading to a worthwhile treatment. When we start trading a lower quality of life for a greater quantity of life, we have entered a zero-sum game that embraces the momentum to treat and results, ultimately, in excessive and futile therapy. Overtreatment at the end of life will, at a minimum, waste some of your precious time and, in the worst case, cause a complication that will shorten your life. Hospice care breaks that momentum by offering an alternative perspective that focuses on maximizing the quality of life while the disease takes its natural course.

Hospice care is an important component of the end-of-life strategy.

It is, in a sense, a medical system that is an alternative to the test-and-treat standard of care that traps the elderly in a perpetual cycle of medicalization. In reality, there is no cure for terminal illnesses, no new beginning for end-stage diseases, and no fountain of youth for the aged. Therefore, cyclically testing and reflexively treating patients in these circumstances can only do harm.

Beyond the principles of caring, "hospice care" is a term that conflates a location, a philosophy, a treatment program, and a regulatory algorithm under a single rubric. Confusion abounds when patients, family members, and medical personnel do not specify to which aspect they are referring.

HOSPICE AS A PLACE: FROM CHURCH TO HOSPITAL TO HOME

The existence of hospice care dates back to the eleventh century. In the ancient Roman Catholic tradition, churches offered havens for weary travelers and pilgrims. Many of the pilgrims were sick or wounded as they made their pilgrimage to the holy site of their choice. The fusion of spiritual care and nursing care started here. Ultimately, as expertise in a traveler's respite care developed, and in the absence of hospitals, these havens became the focus of care for the terminally ill or incurables.

Independent of religious travels, the concept of centers of care exclusively for the terminally ill dates back to the seventeenth century. As the science of medicine developed and concentrated patients in hospitals during the eighteenth and nineteenth centuries, churches began sharing the care of the terminally ill. With the development of modern medicine in the early twentieth century, and the medicalization of death in the mid-twentieth century, the role of the church in the care of the terminally ill was diminished. During the second half of the twentieth century, most patients in the Western world were, therefore, dying in hospitals.

Modern hospice care began in England during the 1950s. Dame Cicely Saunders created the modern hospice philosophy of treating the patient's physical and emotional needs and not the patient's illness.[1] Initially this began in stand-alone hospices. Again, these were frequently associated with church groups or church facilities. Finally, as hospice treatments were refined and equipment became more portable, hospice care began to move out of facilities and into the patients' homes.

Currently, most hospice patients in America are treated at home.[2] However, hospice care can be delivered in hospitals, nursing homes, or stand-alone hospice facilities. The term "in hospice" used to mean a physical place. Now it means a concept of care delivered wherever the patient's needs dictate. Patients can move back and forth freely as their clinical situation changes and circumstances demand. Most patients prefer hospice care at home, but some prefer to be in a hospice facility or a nursing home with hospice support.[3]

"Respite care" for the caretakers is another example of when a patient might move to an inpatient facility. The burden of caretaking on family, friends, and relatives is heavy. Occasionally they need a break to recharge their own batteries. Under these circumstances the patient can leave home and spend a variable number of days in a facility while the family and caretakers take a break.

HOSPICE AS A PHILOSOPHY

The crux of Dame Saunders's philosophy of care was to separate the goal of curing an incurable illness, or the intent of extending life at all cost, from the desire to manage symptoms. Hospice as a philosophy has become more nuanced over time. Although narcotics and tranquilizers remain the foundation of most treatments, hospice care can now include other palliative modalities that border on what appear to be attempts at treatment. As long as quality is emphasized over quantity of life and the proposed palliative therapy is designed to diminish symptoms for someone who is not actively dying, what appears to be aggressive therapy can be considered.[4]

HOSPICE AS A TREATMENT PROGRAM

Hospice care varies from patient to patient, depending on clinical factors such as diagnosis, age, and secondary illnesses. Cardio-respiratory illnesses are sure to be treated with an emphasis on oxygenation, water pills, and bronchodilators. Neurological illnesses will be treated with an emphasis on maintaining movement and flexibility. Cancer complications will be addressed individually; seizures will be treated with drugs, bone pain will be treated with opiates and radiation, diarrhea will be treated with medications and antibiotics, and a program to prevent constipation will be instituted.

There is no limit to treatment options as long as they are palliative, not life-prolonging, in intent. However, pain control and anxiety control are the central focus of most treatment plans. Physical pain is treated with a variety of medications, including opiates. Emotional pain is treated with spiritual or psychological support, tranquilizers, and psychiatric medications as indicated. Spiritual pain is addressed by pastoral care.

As performance status declines, the complications of prolonged bed rest become almost universal. Skin care and the prevention of skin breakdown are emphasized. An air mattress will be supplied. Bowel habits will be closely monitored to prevent the complications of constipation (a fecal impaction).

Steroids are given to suppress inflammation. Antibiotics can be added to control the discomfort of certain infections or can be declined to hasten death (e.g., in the case of pneumonia or sepsis).

Hospice providers supply mechanical devices intended to improve the quality of life. Wheelchairs, commode chairs, lift devices, bedside tables, urinals, bedpans, catheters, diapers, and other things improve quality of life and prevent complications. Hospital beds help patients and caregivers. Variable flow air mattresses prevent bedsores. Mechanical lifts help patients from bed to chair and delay the bed-bound status. Condom catheters and diapers limit transfers, and limiting transfers limits opportunities to fall.

Mechanical devices that prolong life (ventilators and defibrillators, for example) would be inconsistent with hospice philosophy. These might be continued if already in place when the patient chose to enter hospice and if a plan to deactivate them has been established.

HOSPICE AS A REGULATORY CONCEPT

Getting accepted into hospice care is to navigate a regulatory obstacle course. In principle, a person should be able to choose to enter hospice care at any time, by accepting the hospice philosophy and establishing a way to pay for the services. In practice, most people rely on the government (or an insurance plan) to pay for it, and many regulations are the result. Because people tend to delay admission as long as possible and because the vast majority of hospice care is paid for by Medicare, entering hospice and being eligible for hospice benefits have become virtually synonymous. In other words, the medical benefits of hospice are confused and conflated with the financial benefits paid for by the government.

In reality this plays out as an issue when one is trying to get admitted to a hospice program early in the course of one's terminal illness.

The medical and emotional benefits of hospice care are optimized the longer one is in such a program. But the financial Medicare payments ("benefits") are limited to patients who have been "certified," by a physician, to have a life expectancy of less than six months. From the government perspective this is a common-sense regulation designed to limit excessive and indefinite spending. From the patient's perspective it discourages early admission. From the doctor's point of view, it is a lot easier to predict the future and to certify that a patient has less than six months to live when they are, in fact, at death's door with one week to live than it is when they might use the maximum government allowance of a six-month life expectancy.

To be clear, Medicare recognizes that it is impossible to accurately predict the disease course for a particular patient. It is harder still to look at a diagnosis and the clinical parameters of a particular patient and estimate that in six months 51 percent of patients in similar circumstances will be dead. But if attempted honestly, it is at that point the doctor can certify that the average life expectancy for a group of patients with these clinical parameters is less than six months. Of course, in this scenario, when six months has passed, if the patient is proven to be in the lucky 49 percent of survivors, some accommodation must be made. In this case, the government allows recertification for another six months of hospice care.

As a physician, I had several patients who signed up early for hospice care and, having survived more than six months, received federal benefits for a second or third set of six months. Individual doctors are not punished for the occasional success story when a patient survives longer than expected. Most patients can be readmitted for an additional six months without issue. Where doctors and organizations have an institutionalized pattern of fraudulent certification, then problems arise and federal regulators sanction them. But this is the providers' problem, not yours.

CONFLATION OF HOSPICE CARE TERMINOLOGY CAUSES CONFUSION

Given the meanings (location, philosophy, treatment plan, and regulatory requirements) that the terms "hospice care" or "in hospice" conjure up, it is important to clarify the usage in every particular case. I have been party to countless conversations in which a nurse, doctor, or family want to talk about "going into hospice" (meaning they want to discuss the hospice philosophy) and the patient replies, "I don't want to go anywhere, I just want to go home." I have also been party to conversations where a patient wants to discuss the benefits of hospice (again a philosophical or clinical discussion) and the hospice intake coordinator replies, "The government won't pay for that, you're not ready for hospice." That was the case when I wanted my father to consider an application to hospice.

Two experienced nurses saw regulatory obstacles and preferred not to engage in a discussion that they thought would confuse him.

Therefore, whenever these terms are used, significant aggravation can be saved if the participants are clear on which meaning is being invoked.

MY FATHER'S HOSPICE EXPERIENCE

My father's ambivalence about hospice care began with my mother's illness. When she signed DNR papers, he kept them tucked away in a file. He hid her DNR bracelet in his wallet. He did not want to face the facts.

When she had her interview for hospice he was cool. Advanced lung cancer is a straightforward admission. When she was accepted he was aloof. When hospice representatives came to discuss the practicalities of medical equipment and medications, he felt they were an intrusion. He did not want their emotional or spiritual support. He felt that they offered little daily assistance. He could not see what he was getting. He could not visualize their benefits. He did not understand what they did or what they had to offer. It was not for lack of attempts at communication, but for unwillingness on his part to hear. He thought that they did "nothing."

Indeed, my mother's decline was comparatively swift and uneventful. After taking one or two courses of low-dose chemotherapy in the months after her diagnosis, and at my firm suggestion, she signed up for hospice and attended her granddaughter's wedding that May, in Washington, DC.

The trip went off without a hitch. My father arranged most all of that. She was wheeled in and out of events in her wheelchair. The handicapped room in the hotel was a success. He did not have any sense that her hospice played any role in the success of the wedding. It did, in fact, though indirectly.

As the father of the bride I had plenty to be concerned about. My mother's health was one of my biggest concerns. What if she became short of breath? What if she tripped in the hotel room and needed pain medications? What if something worse happened? How could we keep her out of the emergency room or hospital?

Well, hospice care is transportable. Because of her hospice status in Milwaukee we were able to obtain local hospice contacts and hospice status in DC. If she had had a medical crisis in DC, it would have complicated the wedding, but we would not have lost control of her care. With her papers in hand and hospice nurses just a phone call away, she could have avoided or finessed most excessive emergency treatments. Oxygen, limited medical supplies, and pain medications could have been brought to the hotel. If she needed hospitalization, it would have been on a ward with a hospice bed. Her care was one anxiety I could set aside, although at the time its contingencies were beyond my father's grasp.

They returned to Milwaukee and had a drama-free summer from the medical perspective. I visited them in September. Mom was still sitting up in the living room during the day, eating at the table for most meals, and sleeping in her own bed. A few days after our departure, she started to fade. The hospice provided all the necessary equipment, and she died a week later.

Because my father could care for most of her needs right up to the end, the benefits of the hospice were not apparent to him until the last week. But they were apparent to me because I knew what could go wrong and how they could have helped if circumstances arose.

At some point, after my mother's death, Dad started wearing her DNR bracelet. It was not an officially condoned act but it was an emotional act of loyalty and personal intent. It was a declaration that he was done with reflexive, aggressive medical care.

A few months after his ninety-third birthday, when I saw that he was progressively becoming a danger to himself, I began to explore the potential for his admission to a home hospice. Keep in mind, my mother's diagnosis of advanced lung cancer was an automatic admission ticket to hospice. My father's declining performance status was not, and the Visiting Nurse Association's hospice refused to admit him because his lymphoma was inactive and he left the apartment once per month.[5]

Frustrated with that response, I asked the nurse manager of Dad's home care team to explore other options, and she invited a for-profit hospice organization to visit and interview him. They admitted him the next week, opining that a lymphoma was a cancer and that escaping the apartment for a symphony or opera was a quality-of-life issue that they could support. "I have matriculated," he said on the phone, and I can imagine his dismissive hand wave.

My father's relationship with his own hospice care began as it had ended with my mother's. He was passively defiant and refused to acknowledge that in the absence of a medical crisis they were earning their federal subsidy. He did not want to talk about minor medical problems. He simply dismissed them as tolerable. He preferred not to talk directly about death or major medical problems but did so begrudgingly because he found those discussions to be better than patronizing, euphemistic circumlocutions. He did not want their spiritual or emotional support.

Within twenty-four hours of his admission, the hospice had produced an upgraded hospital bed, some new toilet appliances, an oxygen tank, and a "comfort kit." They took over his medication purchasing, sorting, and distribution. They arranged for supplemental physical therapy, nursing visits, and bed baths. They replaced his anti–bed sore air mattress with an upgrade. Months later in the course of his decline, they provided a bed-to-chair hoist.

He complained about the presence of the oxygen tank, regulator, and mask. "I don't need it, I don't want to pay for it, and I don't want the government to pay for it," he complained. I explained that he might need it and that the government was happy to pay for it because it might keep him out of the emergency room. If and when he did need it, he would not want to wait, breathless for hours, pending delivery. It gave me comfort knowing it was there. He should have been pleased. Instead, to keep him relaxed, we moved the oxygen to another room, out of his sight line.

The "comfort kit" was a small plastic box to be placed in the refrigerator. It contained multiple medications, most of them "controlled substances." It was sealed to prevent tampering and was labeled, "Do Not Open without Instructions of the Hospice Doctor or Nurse." Its contents would have included an opiate, various other pain medications, something for seizures, powerful medications for nausea and vomiting, tranquilizers, and sleeping pills. Most of the medications were present in a form that could be given by mouth, under the tongue, or rectally as a suppository. This way, in the event of an emergency, a family member or non-medical caregiver could deliver the initial dose of medication under the instructions of the hospice professional while arrangements for an urgent home evaluation were made.

Dad never verbalized a concern about a new-onset seizure, unexplained vomiting, new-onset pain, shortness of breath, hallucinations, or panic attacks, but their potential haunted me. In the absence of hospice care and a comfort kit, any such occurrence could precipitate a 911 call and an ER visit that could spin out of control. Dad did live in constant fear of falling and the subsequent pain from such trauma. The medication kit made immediately available the first dose of morphine that could mean so much.

He never warmed up to his hospice nurses. They are, indeed, a special breed of person. The work they do is admirable. They are in the awkward situation of constantly dealing with the practicalities of death and dying. There is the associated risk of giving offense for being too brusque or not blunt enough. Their patients are, by definition, going to die under their care and supervision. One moment they might be chatting pleasantly about some mundane scheduling detail and the next moment they would have to discuss the characteristics of a death rattle and how to distinguish it from a coughing spell. It is a difficult balance to maintain.

Most patients benefit by some degree of spiritual support supplied by a hospice team. My father did not. Dad had no spiritual resources other than great literature. He had never been to church as a child or young adult. He had no religious training. He did not believe in heaven. He did not expect to see my mother on "the other side." He declined the spiritual offerings of the hospice team and refused to see their non-denominational pastors. He was comfortable reviewing the humanistic lessons of great literary and great historical works. His caregivers and his family comforted him.

It is impossible to be all things to all people. To the degree that hospice care is a service industry, they are bound to fail some patients, and there is no second chance for service "recovery." To the degree that hospice care is a medical profession, hospice nurses have an enormous amount to offer. Ultimately my father accepted them as professionals.

Although Dad never embraced all aspects of hospice care, he came to appreciate much of it. There was the "in your face" weekly visit when he had to confront his mortality with the hospice nurse. He did not look forward to that. There was the medical equipment about which he was ambivalent, but ultimately grateful. There was the comfort kit, which he never needed but the importance of which he could intellectually understand. And there were multiple little niceties in terms of procuring medical supplies (diapers, bed pads, urinals, catheters, leg bags, bandages, medications, etc.) that freed up his staff for more personal time with him and his apartment.

As a physician, I knew some of the crises that could have befallen him. I could imagine any number of problems that, absent the hospice presence, would have resulted in trips to the ER and hospital where well-intentioned medical experts would overdiagnose, overtreat, and overcommit to follow-up. With the hospice presence we had an opportunity in place to forestall the vast majority of those crises. Blessed are the frail elderly who do not have to visit the emergency room. In that regard, my father was blessed.

UNDERSTANDING AND ACCEPTING THE BENEFITS OF HOSPICE CARE

Accepting hospice and getting accepted into it are two different things. The first is a philosophical decision and the second is a provider decision. Understanding the medical and emotional benefits of hospice care is distinct from understanding the financial benefits as paid to your provider by the federal government.

Getting a patient and a family to accept hospice care requires early and regular attention. Avoiding the subject postpones the benefit of hospice care without delaying the inevitability of needing it. Promoting it early and often may be uncomfortable, but the worst thing is to wait until it is too late and to die in the hospital or to transfer out of the hospital with only a few days of compromised existence remaining.

Most hospice proponents believe that it takes three months of hospice care to maximize its clinical (medical and psychological) benefits. Unfortunately, consideration given to hospice care is so regularly delayed that the median survival is barely over a month. In one study, 15 percent of patients died within seven days and 28 percent died within fourteen days.[6]

The benefits of hospice should be described as the emotional and physical comfort of dying at home, surrounded by the familiar, and with control over as many factors as possible. Admission before the distractions of a final medical crisis allows families the opportunity to value one another and the possibility of repairing frayed relationships. That may not sound like much, but it should be contrasted with the unpleasantness of death in a hospital without personal effects or memories and subject to the whims, misunderstandings, isolation, and regulations of a team of doctors, nurses, technicians, and orderlies.

A good exercise in that perspective is for all caregivers and family members to seek every opportunity to visit a hospital or nursing home and to observe the hustle and bustle of care there. In such a place you are likely to see disoriented, despondent, and confused patients "sundowning." This phenomenon of anguished confusion occurs regularly among the elderly, most commonly when deprived of familiar home surroundings, and it is most evident when the evening shift is preparing to leave and the less well-staffed night shift arrives. The sundowning patients are routinely left in their recliners in the hall, restraints in place, beseeching the ebbing and flowing staff to "help," "get a doctor," or "call my family."

One way of introducing the concept of hospice care is to introduce its first cousin, palliative care, as soon as a serious illness is identified.[7] The old model of health care consisted of life-prolonging care with the intent to cure until overtreatment becomes futile and imminent death undeniable. Then the unpleasant conversation about death and hospice care tends to be weighty and late. Now, palliative care specialists are available well before end-of-life care is needed. They can help with the control of symptoms associated with serious illness such as diarrhea, constipation, shortness of breath, anxiety, itching, and, of course, pain. Not only do patients do better with months or years of palliative care but they tend to enter hospice earlier in the course of their illness with improved quality of life throughout.

Another barrier to accepting hospice care is the emotional roller coaster of illness. The daily fluctuations of emotional and physical strength prompt a willingness to consider hospice when feeling low and dismissing it when feeling better. The broader trajectory of illness is forgotten as patients adapt to their reduced capacities. Watching a patient limp toward the decision is a process of fits and starts. When depressed by new symptoms a patient will embrace the process. When adjusted to a new, reduced performance status they will be optimistic and shy away from accepting their mortality.

Caregivers and family members will resonate with this temporary optimism and they will amplify it. "Oh, he's not ready for hospice, he's not ready to give up." This practice simply delays the inevitable to the detriment of all. Rather than enjoying the fresh optimism in the sense of a good day, or the best possible day, in a series of difficult days, a good day is assumed to be a sign to continue hoping for better.

People are fickle. Disease is not rational. Sometimes people will want to be in hospice in a general sense but want to enjoy some treatment that seems inconsistent with the hospice philosophy. My father wanted to stop taking his medications. Because they were standard anti-hypertensives and a statin for lowering cholesterol, we could expect no dramatic turn for the worse, but the intention was clear. He was sending a signal that he wanted to hasten his death.

Simultaneously he wanted a flu vaccination. He was not afraid to choose to die, but he did not want to be "sick."

Inconsistency is not a reason to defer hospice admission, reject a candidate, or downplay the benefits. The hospice philosophy is flexible enough on small things to rationalize minor treatments as comforting if they improve the patient's quality of life either physically or emotionally.

One of the most overlooked benefits of hospice care is its transportability as described by my mother's trip to my daughter's wedding.

Another benefit of hospice care, unclear to the uninitiated, is the elimination of unnecessary doctor visits. These usually result in diagnostic tests and a tendency for follow-up tests or visits. An example of this occurred when my father developed itching without a rash. Nothing had changed in terms of his diet, detergent, soap, or lotions for months. When a short course of Benadryl and steroids did not permanently resolve the symptoms, his primary care doctor, untrained in the ways of hospice care, advised that he better come in for a checkup. This would have resulted in blood tests, possible X-rays, and follow-up of abnormal results as the doctor worked through her checklist of potential diagnoses that cause itching.

His hospice nurse spoke for all of us when she responded, "That's not going to happen!" The primary care physician was clearly well-intentioned but misguided. She was focused on a diagnosis not a symptom. We did not care about a new diagnosis anymore. We turned to the hospice doctor, who prescribed high-dose steroids as needed.

There is an understandable and unavoidable tension in the process of accepting hospice care. That tension exists at multiple levels. Doctors must relate to patients in such a way as to find the sweet spot for encouraging admission. Doctors must understand the Medicare requirements for a patient to be accepted. The hospice of choice must understand the regulatory requirements so as to be in compliance with the law when accepting a patient for admission. And regulators must be able to discern legitimate requests for hospice care from fraudulent abuse of the hospice system.

Like many health care delivery services, hospices can be divided into nonprofit and for-profit enterprises. It is pertinent to be aware of this distinction. I generally prefer nonprofit enterprises. I believe nonprofit hospitals, home-care services, and hospices are slightly more mission driven than for-profit organizations. But make no mistake: the challenge of keeping a nonprofit organization open in this era of reduced reimbursement can spawn the same kind of misjudgments that inspire profit-making groups to bend rules for the shareholders. You have to evaluate your hospice options individually.

HOSPICE "CARE": WHAT ARE ITS PARAMETERS?

Hospice "care" is not routine, daily, unskilled nursing care. It is not home health aide care. Except in emergencies, hospice "care" can be hard to discern. For the patient admitted early in the course of their final decline, hospice "care" is invisible. The hospice nurse visits once a week, organizes the pillbox, updates their assessment, and schedules a return visit. Many family members are disappointed by these facts. They think that when a patient signs on to hospice care they will get a care team to take over. They expect to do less and have more assistance. In fact, they, the family, will continue to have the responsibility for supplying or hiring most of the home health aide care.

What hospice care does supply are supervision, training, equipment, medical supplies, respite care, travel coverage, twenty-four-hour phone consultations, a few hours of nursing assistance per week, and emergency skilled nursing care.

I have already commented on the arrival of a hospital bed, oxygen tank, and comfort kit immediately upon admission. Deliveries of diapers, catheter-related supplies, and prescription medicines occur throughout the admission. Later, as decline progresses, some hospices supply occasional home health services such as a bed bath, once or twice a week. Later still, when a patient starts to "actively die," hospice nurse visits occur more frequently to adjust medications and counsel the family. If all goes well, hospice care can look quite detached from day to day "caring."

It is when things do not go well that the benefits of hospice are most apparent. To the family members with health care backgrounds, those who know what can go wrong and who are devoted to avoiding the medicalization of death, knowing that hospice is in the background is a great comfort.

For example, on a mundane level, the risk of falling at home exists until a patient becomes bed-bound. Every transfer from bed to wheelchair (or commode) and back risks an injurious fall; at a minimum every transfer risks a slip to the floor from which the patient and a single caregiver cannot easily recover.[8] In the event of a fall or a fall with injury, the caregiver need not call 911. Hospice care can swing into action. The comfort kit can be opened and pain meds supplied. The hospice nurse and lift assistance will come immediately. Lacerations can be sutured. Portable X-rays can be arranged at home. Fractures can be splinted. Most emergency room visits can be avoided or aborted. Overtreatment can be avoided.

On a more sophisticated level, complications of illness that are unforeseen by the caregivers can be addressed by hospice expertise. For example, patients with lung cancer are at risk for brain metastases. Brain metastases frequently cause seizures. There are few things as disquieting as observing one's first seizure, and in that event the temptation to call 911 for emergency care would be intense. In hospice care, the comfort kit is stocked with anticonvulsant suppositories, and a hospice nurse will make an emergency visit.

When skilled nursing is required for some other unforeseen circumstances (pain control, seizure control, IV medications, etc.), the hospice service will supply such care, twenty-four hours per day for up to a week, to control symptoms and avoid hospitalizations.

In the rare circumstance when a patient does need to be transported to an emergency room, a hospice nurse will be dispatched to meet them there and minimize overaggressive treatment. If a patient needs admission to a hospital, the hospital's hospice and palliative care team will be notified.

Finally, when a patient is "actively" dying, many inexplicable manifestations of the process will unsettle the inexperienced caregiver. Shouting out, speaking jibberish, jerking extremities, agonal breathing, and death rattles can be explained, soothed, and treated by hospice experts.

HOSPICE CARE: AN ALTERNATIVE MEDICAL SYSTEM

In summary, hospice care is an alternative medical system that has the potential to liberate patients from the momentum of treatment that ultimately becomes futile treatment. Its doctors and nurses are forward thinking, supplying equipment and medications in advance of possible problems. This aborts the standard test-and-treat practice of reactive medical care, sparing time- and energy-consuming office visits, ER visits, and hospitalizations. It is a system that allows days of good-quality life that would have otherwise been spent in medical waiting rooms, doctors' offices, clinic visits, radiology suites, emergency rooms, or ICUs. Hospice care protects patients with a team of medical professionals whose goal is to improve the day, not fight for another day complicated by side effects of treatments or medications.

Yes, one needs a steely resolve and a clear-eyed view of reality to forego the exaggerated promise of aggressive medical care. But the benefits are measurable. For every day of life gained by aggressive pre-hospice therapy, yet compromised by the side effects and complications of medical treatments, the hospice patient will better enjoy a day of peace and comfort surrounded by friends and family.

Things to Remember/Things to Consider

- When thinking about hospice, keep separate and clear the confusion of place, philosophy, care plan, admission criteria, clinical benefits, and financial benefits.
- Hospice does little home health care and supplies nursing care only as needed.
- Hospice is your best protection from CPR and overtreatment.
- Getting admitted early maximizes the clinical benefits.
- Hospice care is transportable and renewable.
- If you live more than six months in hospice care, that is not your problem; that is their problem.

Chapter Twelve

Voluntary Refusal of Fluid and Food

Life is pleasant. Death is peaceful. It's the transition that's troublesome.

—Isaac Asimov

T HIS BOOK IS about looking at the course of an illness and recognizing realistic milestones. At the very end of life one such milestone is the realization that further medical treatment is futile, some combination of symptoms and diminished performance status is intolerable, and death is inevitable. And then, when nothing can be done to add quality to existence, death might still seem too far off. At this point, feeling powerless but seeking control, some people do choose to look at ways to hasten death.

This chapter is not about suicide, assisted suicide, medical aid in dying, or terminal sedation.[1] Where medical aid in dying is available (currently that is limited to California, Colorado, Montana, Oregon, Vermont, Washington, and the District of Columbia), it should be considered. But in those same states, and in the majority of states where medical aid in dying is not available, the refusal of fluid and food is an effective and ethical option available to all terminally ill patients. Such action isn't taken lightly—in fact, it is frequently discussed but much less commonly pursued. However, toward the end of life, everyone should be aware of this option.

It is difficult to put into lay terms when you should consider this action. Too frequently it is thought of as simply "giving up." Yet for a thoughtful elderly patient who has studied their disease course, is in a hospice setting, and who feels powerless and reliant on others, the conscious action of refusing to eat and drink should be understood. Not only does this decision put the patient back in charge of the moment, it demonstrates a staunch independence that proves the time is right and the time has come, overshadowing the ambivalence some associate with the assistance required of the "suicide pill."

There are multiple dizzying medical terms to describe the act of death by self-dehydration. The resultant alphabet soup of acronyms is off-putting. The term currently gaining the most traction is voluntarily stopping eating and drinking, or VSED. Its appeal is derived from its descriptive simplicity and the ability to pronounce the acronym as a word (pronounced *VEESed*). Like most of the other terms and acronyms, VSED wrongly places the emphasis on declining food. Death is by dehydration, not starvation, and that is one reason why I prefer to avoid the acronyms. I prefer the terms "terminal dehydration" and "self-dehydration" because they emphasize the power of the choice and the physiology of the process.

PRACTICAL, ETHICAL, AND LEGAL ASPECTS OF REFUSING FLUID AND FOOD

Terminal dehydration sounds grim, I admit. Most people think it sounds, at least, very uncomfortable. My father could not get past his concept that starvation was involved; yet the facts are otherwise. Most hospice nurses describe death by refusing to drink and eat as preferable to death by physician-assisted suicide.[2] I will give details when I discuss the physiology of the process.

More important, self-dehydration avoids the ethical quandaries some see in the concept of assisted suicide, as well as the moral conflicts created by actual suicide. Whether refusing to drink and eat at the end of life is a variation on suicide has been debated for decades. These debates have come to a practical conclusion, however, because the national hospice organizations have accepted the practice as an ethical one, and the federal courts have declined to take a position against it.

Most important, when the status quo is intolerable because of disease and advanced age, death by dehydration works effectively to alleviate suffering, empower the patient, and unburden the caregivers. All of these are attributes of a good death.

In the absence of intractable pain, in which case medical aid in dying or terminal sedation might be preferable, terminal dehydration is the best resolution to the problems of creating a good death because it requires a combination of disease, debility, and willful intention to institute. The decision initially inspires confidence because the patient is back in control. This confidence is amplified by the mild euphoria of caloric withdrawal. In the vast majority of cases, that euphoria gently progresses to a clouded sensorium, sleepiness, and coma.

DEHYDRATION AS PART OF A NATURAL DEATH

I became aware of self-dehydration while serving on the board of a hospice. At that time, many of the principles that I just set forth were still being debated in hospitals, nursing homes, and the courts, but they were being practiced in enlightened private homes and hospices. As a physician, I had observed many hospital deaths. My experience was that those deaths involved the last attempt at staving off a terminal illness, including the pain and anguish of unnecessary medicalization, followed by a phase of physical and mental depletion. During this phase of advanced exhaustion, the natural inability to eat became paramount. Families became anxious and protective. "How can my loved one recover if he can't eat?" was a common entreaty.

If the patient or agent came to understand that recovery was not possible and they accepted counseling to withdraw intravenous fluid and artificial nutrition (tube feeding or intravenous feeding), based on the understanding that further treatment was futile and selectively feeding the disease process, then the process of dehydration had begun, not by design so much as by default. In the absence of hydration and calories, most patients will die in six to ten days, and 85 percent will have passed away quietly within two weeks.

In the hospice setting, I was observing that if a patient had voluntarily declined that "last heroic treatment," a conversation about terminal dehydration was more easily undertaken. I further noted that these patients avoided weeks of pain and suffering compared to hospitalized patients.

That is why one article in the *New England Journal of Medicine* resonated with me so strongly (see endnote 3 in chapter 7 or endnote 2 in this chapter). It described the generally positive observations of nurses dealing with hospice patients in the process of hastening death by refusing fluid and food. My thoughts at the time were that the practice added a willful and voluntary component to the natural process of death that I had observed to take place involuntarily and tardily in hospitalized patients. Having embraced it, I have seen it serve successfully as a technique to initiate and then control the final chapter in many lives.

The refusal of fluid and food is a phase that is common to every slow death. To the untrained observer, it may not be perceived to be such a phase as a person involuntarily fades, but on every deathbed there is a period of time when the patient is too weak to eat, then too weak to drink, and then too weak to breathe. Death arrives voluntarily or involuntarily. Self-dehydration alters the time frame of a natural process just enough to spare needless suffering but not enough to be practically confused with a premature death, an impulsive act, or suicide.

MY FATHER AND THE REFUSAL OF FLUID AND FOOD

Curiously, my father was unable to embrace terminal dehydration although he had incorporated the concept into his living will. At my suggestion, that document contained a clause that allowed him to choose not to be manually fed and referenced the *New England Journal of Medicine* article about nurses' observations of the practice. We discussed it intermittently as an exit strategy. And while he understood the practice intellectually, he never really considered it. Despite his advanced debility, his appetite remained robust, and he enjoyed his meals too much to consider giving them up.

About a month after his admission to hospice care, I made a routine visit. He was living a bed-to-chair existence. He was tolerating but lamenting the degradations that old age was visiting on him. "I have lived too long," he said upon my arrival.

I raised the topic of exit strategies. I likened voluntary dehydration to his law school classmate's decision to stop hemodialysis two years before this visit. Dad's mind wandered to his classmate's choice to "pull that plug." He had not emotionally connected with it at the time, but he wished he had such a mechanical option to exercise as we spoke. Then Dad changed the subject.

Two months later, when my wife, Debbie, and I made our Christmas visit, I outlined again the exit strategy of refusing to drink and eat. It may have seemed particularly incongruous to be planning our holiday menu during one conversation and discussing voluntary dehydration during the next, but there was a reason behind this. These discussions can be awkward. They can be hard. In every situation, the patient will be weak and frail compared to the advisor. The discussion, therefore, is asymmetrical. In my case, as a doctor with experience and opinions on the subject of exit strategies, the discussion was even more asymmetrical, and my father might have felt I was forcing the issue. I hoped that by reviewing the concept of self-dehydration while planning Christmas dinner, I signaled that such decisions would be his alone and could be delayed until well after we left.

Again, Dad listened and asked a few questions about "starving." I repeated that when people felt the time was right to invoke this plan, their appetite was already gone. Just as the flu, at its worst, suppresses our appetite, most patients with advanced illnesses lose interest in eating. I explained that disease and debility had generally taken these patients past the point of a metabolism that matched intake with output to a condition known as catabolism (burning more calories than ingested). I told him that with end-stage cancer, heart failure, or lung disease, a disproportionate number of calories are burned and the appetite is greatly reduced. At this point refusing to eat and drink simply accelerates the process.

Any minor hunger pains that occur will be rapidly dissipated by the euphoria of fasting and the sense of taking control. This euphoria is generally replaced by the sleepiness of dehydration in a few days. Coma and death follow comparatively quietly. But because meals continued to give him pleasure, he was not ready. Sometime later, he might reach that point, I thought.

During that particular conversation, my dad changed the exit strategy discussion to one of eliminating his non-palliative prescription medications. It was clear that he was still not ready to consider self-dehydration. One day later, he kissed us goodbye, saying, "This has been our last Christmas." The next day he stopped his medications. He wanted to take steps, but he could only go so far.

THE PHYSIOLOGY OF REFUSING TO DRINK AND EAT

The process of hastening death by refusing to eat and drink is simple and the physiology straightforward. When the patient is interested and educated, they pick a time and date to decline food and fluid. The absence of fat and carbohydrate calories stimulates protein metabolism in twenty-four to forty-eight hours. This, in turn, creates ketosis (the accumulation of ketones—a toxic metabolite) and a sense of euphoria that rapidly displaces most sensations of hunger. The absence of water intake concentrates the build-up of metabolic toxins and amplifies the effects of renal insufficiency (kidney failure). After a few days, sleepiness progresses to a coma, the process of actively dying is initiated, and ultimately a painless disturbance of the heart's rhythm ends the process. This is death by dehydration.

Most studies show that two thirds of patients have no complaints of hunger at all. One third of patients have transient hunger pains. A small minority has persistent hunger symptoms. These can be managed with narcotics and sedatives.

Similarly, one third of patients have no thirst problems. One third of patients have transient thirst problems, and the remaining third of patients use moist swabs or towels to manage complaints of a dry mouth.

Dehydration, itself, is painless. Unfortunately, natural death, with or without dehydration, is not always smooth and serene; no death is guaranteed to be smooth and serene. Natural death is never fast enough to satisfy every observer. Respiratory patterns change. The nervous system, although suppressed by coma, shuts down in fits and starts. The process can be misunderstood and mischaracterized, even by health care professionals.

In the case of my father, one of the certified nursing assistants supplied by the hospice proved savvy enough to accurately predict his death one month in advance of the event, but she also referred to "the pain of dehydration," confusing my older sister, who was with him during his last few days. This is a common misconception. What the nursing assistant was referring to as the "pain of dehydration" was the bizarre, inexplicable, and unsettling behavior of patients who are actively dying.

Compounding this misunderstanding is the frequent use of morphine for end-of-life symptoms. Known as a pain medicine, it is also used for respiratory distress (to relieve the "air hunger" of pneumonia), to augment medications that relieve anxiety, and for its euphoric effect. Therefore, the use of morphine should not always be interpreted as indicative of the presence of pain.

Furthermore, the deathbed scene is impossible to predict. It can be serene for periods of time. It can be dominated by periods of delirium. It can be punctuated by inexplicable behavior that invites overinterpretation. Many patients vocalize nonsensically. Immigrant patients may revert to the language of their childhood after decades of non-use. My sister reports that my father called out for his mother. What was he thinking? Some patients will grunt or twitch. Others will clutch at the air. Limbs spasm. Throats close. Sphincters relax. Bowels open. The process can be unpleasant to observe. Most of these behaviors are manifestations of neurological "shutdown." They also occur in patients who are dying in the hospital and receiving intravenous fluids to prevent dehydration, at their family's request. Most doctors advise that intravenous fluids only delay the inevitable and agree that simple dehydration does not cause pain.

Make no mistake, all of these perplexing symptoms can, and occasionally do, occur during death by asphyxiation from drug overdose, the most common form of medical aid in dying. Nausea, vomiting, aspiration, choking, and suffocation can also occur with drug overdoses, diminishing the "dignity" of this death.

It is our habit to interpret, perhaps overinterpret, these deathbed behaviors. No one can divine their provenance or meaning. One small comfort for those of us encouraging or undertaking death by dehydration is to understand and appreciate that "natural death" is natural and that dying while attached to a machine is not.

TERMINAL DEHYDRATION: HOW LONG DOES IT LAST?

Patients who refuse fluid and food expire at different times because they start the process with different physiologic foundations. Most patients are euphoric for a day or two and then slip in and out of consciousness. Many are dead in six to ten days. Eighty-five percent are dead within two weeks. It is rare to survive four weeks, and even rarer to survive six. Regardless of how long it takes, somnolence and coma are present most of the time from four to six days until death.

Factors that contribute to a longer than expected clinical course relate to the nutritional status of the patient and the underlying disease process. A well-nourished patient with adequate fat stores will take a day or two more to achieve full protein catabolism, and the presence of retained fluid might slow down the dehydration. On the other hand, a catabolic illness, such as cancer, which consumes calories independent of the patient's baseline metabolism, will shorten the final process. Therefore, a malnourished, dehydrated, thin cancer patient is likely to die in six to ten days, whereas a well-nourished, well-hydrated patient with advanced Parkinson's disease and the crippling pain of a collapsed spine is more likely to be in the small group of patients who survive more than two weeks.

When my father advanced to the stage where he could no longer chew food or swallow liquids safely, he was still able to communicate with single-word expressions. But once choking occurred with each mouthful, with the support of his living will and with the common sense wrought from experience, his professional caregivers declined to force-feed him. He did not ask for more. He had reached the point of passively declining food and fluid. He died four days later.

TIMING THE INITIATION OF SELF-DEHYDRATION

The inability to eat and drink is a phase common to every slow death and to every natural death. When a terminal patient is so depleted by disease and treatment that they reach the natural point where they can no longer nourish themselves or willingly be nourished by mouth, then, like my father, they have backed themselves into the passive decision to refuse food and fluid. Self-dehydration is the active initiation of that final phase by a person educated in its benefits and aware of its consequences before it is forced on them.

The time to take this step varies from patient to patient. It is determined by each patient's balance of debility and commitment. The loss of appetite is common to the end stage of almost every chronic illness. It is a natural dysfunction of the process of dying. Commencing terminal dehydration is an active attempt to foreshorten the process by starting it earlier and speeding it along. But few people start before they are ready, and those who do can change their mind.

Most people fear that starvation is painful. I assume it is when imposed on the healthy and unwilling, as in the case of famine, poverty, and abuse. However, it is not painful at the end of life. Understanding this makes the decision possible but does not determine where the scales of debility and commitment will intersect. If it sounds hard, then you are not ready to refuse fluid and food. If it seems possible and the alternative is intolerable, then you are ready.

My father was never ready to give up food. In this he was not unique. The majority of people who include a self-dehydration clause in their advance directive never act on it.

In the months after my Christmas visit, I visited several times. The subject did not come up again. When I visited in early April, he did not look well. His fine motor skills had deteriorated. "I never thought it would be so hard to die" was the first thing he said on my arrival. "This will be our last visit" was his final statement upon my departure.

HAND-FEEDING: LOVE, BASIC CARE, OR UNINVITED TREATMENT

There is no federal standard regarding manual feeding, but there is state-to-state variation, and it is important to know how your state or jurisdiction views this.

Some states define manual feeding as basic nursing care that must be offered—although, practically speaking, it cannot be forced. Other states perceive of manual feeding as a life-sustaining treatment that can be declined like any other medical treatment under the Patient Self-Determination Act. If your state considers manual feeding to be a sustaining treatment, then it can be withdrawn or withheld without legal implication, even in some institutions. If your state considers it basic care, then the implications are less clear.

In addition to the legal implications, agreeing to observe a patient hasten death by voluntary dehydration and agreeing to withhold such sustenance during the course of that process has emotional implications. Some cultures equate food with care; others equate it with love. Most cultures conflate feeding with caring (in the emotional sense) and basic care (in the nursing sense). At the very end of life, neither of these premises should hold sway, but where does the very end of life begin?

One can be certain the end of life has begun when the body begins shutting down. The appetite is gone, and the ability to chew and swallow is gone. Choking occurs regularly, and therefore people cannot eat. This happens to every patient in every prolonged deathbed scenario. This period of time, when a patient is unable to eat, is variable in length (minutes to days or weeks) but invariable in occurrence. Yet, in most homes, the desire to nurture exists, and the reflex to be sustained survives. The image of a family member offering food is powerful. A patient unable to eat frequently responds with reflexive lip pursing. These actions and images may sustain the caregivers but do nothing for the patient.

At the end of life, too much hand-feeding punishes a patient. That is because putting food into the mouth of someone who is unable to effectively chew and swallow leads to anxiety as the patient rolls the food around the mouth in a cycle of attempted chewing, swallowing, and spitting out. The associated choking increases the risk of aspiration pneumonia. I have seen this scene repeated many times in hospital rooms and nursing homes. It is very discomfiting to watch and, ultimately, the patient is not ingesting enough calories to justify the struggle or the risk.

ACTIVELY DYING PREEMPTS HASTENING DEATH

Dad began to die "actively" one Monday in late April. The hospice nurses had been visiting daily with more frequent adjustments of pain meds and tranquilizers. My older sister was sitting vigil. I was calling her daily to comment on urine output, stool quality, and breathing patterns. I was trying to foresee the end so that she could, too.

On Tuesday morning, we discussed things in general. I asked my sister to ask Dad if he wanted us to stop putting food and fluid to his lips. She didn't want to ask. She was more comfortable letting the scenario play out on its own, albeit very slowly. She did say that the fluid was barely keeping his mouth moist. Perhaps that was her way of saying that withholding fluid didn't have to be formalized.

Our oldest sister was very good to us to have been there. She was quite tough and knew that doing nothing was the best thing to do, but it is extra hard for the uninitiated to withhold food and fluid. However, we were clear that force-feeding was not an option. My sister and I had been prepared to withhold food if Dad ever verbalized that desire, and he had a seasoned cadre of caregivers who stopped offering food and fluid when the risk of choking outweighed the benefits of eating.

Indeed, it was just a few hours later that one of his experienced caregivers turned to my sister and said, "He can't eat anymore; he is choking too much." We had not discussed this specific action with the caregivers. They knew from experience that a natural death was imminent.

The period from the last bite of food and the last sip of fluid to his death was four days. At first, my father was still able to say a few words. However, over the next two days, before he became completely incommunicado, he did not request food or drink.

Dad had steadfastly refused to deny himself food. He enjoyed eating until his very last days. He declined to hasten his death by invoking the voluntary refusal of food and fluid clause in his advance directive. He wanted an exit strategy but did not embrace this one. He enjoyed his meals until the end. On the last day that he could chew, he still commented on his favorite English marmalade. He needed to wait until his altered mental status, based on a mini-stroke or some metabolic change, dimmed his appetite, dampened his taste buds, and damaged his swallowing.

I am confident that if he had voluntarily stopped eating and drinking one week or one month earlier, he would have hastened his death without suffering. But to what end? By this point, he had been ready to die naturally for at least two years; the specific opportunity of a painless infection had just not occurred. He was simply not ready to stop eating before he began the process of actively dying.

PAIN AND HASTENING DEATH

Perhaps a more important factor in Dad's decision making was the absence of intolerable symptoms, the most easily recognized example of which is intractable pain. During his last six months, my father was never in significant pain. That is to say, his life was not ruled by pain. He had aches. He had intermittent pains. He took acetaminophen with codeine (Tylenol 3) regularly. But the pains he had were adequately and easily controlled. Therefore, his life was tolerable. If his minor pains hadn't been controlled or if pain had diminished his quality of life, the decision to hasten the end might have been different.

Of course, pain control is a major focus of hospice care. When possible, it is controlled without medication. Where medication is required, morphine, an analgesic drug that blunts the appetite and suppresses fear, is commonly used. Pain decreases the desire to live, and morphine decreases the desire to eat. The concerns about thirst and hunger are overshadowed by the medications focused on pain control. Those patients with intractable pain at the end of life find it easier to choose death by dehydration than those without. When pain trumps fear, when debility is intolerable, when the end is visible but that horizon is still too distant, then the voluntary refusal of fluid and food is ethical, effective, and acceptable.

SELF-DEHYDRATION: ONE OPTION OFFERING A SENSE OF CONTROL

The goal of this chapter is not to judge the merits of any given exit strategy nor, in particular, to judge the techniques for hastening death. Discontinuing a life-sustaining medication (e.g., insulin) or turning off mechanical assistance (e.g., a defibrillator, hemodialysis, or a left ventricular assist device) are not options for everyone. Where available, medical aid in dying is an important option to consider. It is also important to understand that refusing to drink and eat is universally available, comparable in comfort, and places the process uniquely in the control of the patient.

There is no right time to invoke the concept of terminal dehydration, and those who consider it and do not invoke it are not weak in some way. Rather, the take-home lesson is that self-dehydration is one tool with which to exert some control in a process that is largely out of our control. When the natural process of death is acceptable, the decline is tolerable, the debility accepted, and the end is in sight, the elderly patient might not feel the need to hasten the process. For those who do, voluntary dehydration is a comforting consideration.

Things to Remember/Things to Consider

- In a terminal condition, refusing to eat and drink is a practical, ethical, and legal way to hasten death.
- Refusing to eat and drink results in death by dehydration.
- Dehydration is painless.

Epilogue: Reflections and a Road Map

> When people die, they cannot be replaced. They leave holes that cannot be filled, for it is the fate—the genetic and neural fate—of every human being to be a unique individual, to find his own path, to live his own life, to die his own death.
>
> —Oliver Sacks, MD

IT IS IMPOSSIBLE to describe the scope of human suffering with which medicine deals. The descriptions, in chapters 1 and 5, of typical ICU or post-CPR scenes represent a tiny sample of what modern medicine does to patients in our efforts to deal with illness. When the illness is acute and resolution occurs quickly it is dramatic, gratifying work. When the cure stalls, the disease becomes chronic, and the aggressive treatments are prolonged, the work is draining. But when these violent technologies are imposed on the sick, frail elderly, who have no real chance of long-term survival, it is painful to observe.

When I was in practice and looking at an elderly patient referred for aggressive testing or treatment, I tried to see if that proposed treatment would pass the "mother test": Would I let my mother (or father) undergo it? Frequently, the answer was no. If the patient understood the principles behind that conclusion, they usually accepted the advice with gratitude. One example in which I tried to apply this principle was described in chapter 3, when I recommended that we ignore a flat polyp in the intestine of a frail, old woman.

This book has been aimed at people over the age of sixty-five and the family and friends who care for them. In this book, I do not presume to tell people when to die. I do not pretend that every patient can control every aspect of his or her death. I do not presume to tell readers which doctors to see. I do not presume to tell people what treatments to seek.

Most important, I am not telling elderly patients to decline aggressive treatment arbitrarily. We all know of patients who have enjoyed exceptionally good medical and surgical outcomes at very advanced ages. Unfortunately, they are the exceptions, as we tend to lionize the successes and forget the attempts of those who did not benefit, who suffered complications, or who died trying. So please, if you want to try a complex treatment at an advanced age, proceed with your eyes open, be informed, and have a plan for aggressive passivity in the event of a poor outcome.

I do presume to tell you what I would have told my mother in a given situation. In doing so I am trying to help you organize your thoughts in a different way. I do presume to advise you that every hospitalization and every medical treatment has some degree of unintended consequence, and the degree of damage from those interventions accelerates with age while the degree of benefit is simultaneously reduced. Most important, if you put control of your end-of-life care in the hands of the average physician, you are likely to receive more treatment than is truly beneficial.

At some point every life comes to an end. When one has lived their four score and ten; when one has reached the average life expectancy for their demographic; when one acknowledges a reduced performance status; when one recognizes that they have an illness with a measurable prognosis; then it is easier to create a vision of that eventuality.

For those readers who are blessed with the ability to foresee that endpoint, for those readers who understand that eventually they will be overmastered by their disease or debility, this book should help them find acceptance, assert themselves in the face of overtreatment, and take control of that which can be controlled.

PARADIGM SHIFT: EXAGGERATED PROMISES VERSUS A REALITY CHECK

Whenever a health care article headline starts with the term "Paradigm Shift" you know it will end with breathless optimism. "Paradigm Shift in Cancer Treatment," "Advances in Cardiac Care," "New Paradigm in Alzheimer's Research" are hypothetical examples of articles that will document programs that are interpreted as progress and describe hopeful intentions that are interpreted as promises of a cure. American readers tend to assume that there is always a cure just around the corner, just over the horizon, and, if they hang on long enough, that cure will be theirs.

The paradigm shift we need is a reality check. We need a hard reset of expectations. Medicine has made great progress over the last century. That is a fact. However, another fact is routinely overlooked. Recent progress has been incremental and enormously expensive. Witness the new lung cancer treatments as advertised on television and promising "A Chance to Live Longer" without emphasizing their high costs, serious side effects, and limited benefit.[1] Similarly, future progress will be exponentially expensive, increasingly incremental, and unpredictably dangerous. So when you hear that medical science at the frontiers of terminal illness, advanced age, and human life expectancy "promises" that DNA manipulation and genetic research hold the key to the next great leaps forward, please be skeptical.

COMMERCIALIZATION: INCONSISTENT WITH COMPASSIONATE END-OF-LIFE CARE

More than at any other time, during a patient's advanced years, doctors should remind themselves that medical care is a calling and not a commercial enterprise. But not every physician has your overall interests at heart. Some surgeons will replace joints in patients beyond the point where they can achieve full rehabilitation. Some cardiologists will recommend inserting heart valves when frailty limits full recovery. Some gastroenterologists will stent open digestive tubes that are narrowed by cancer to "buy some time" even though the cancer is growing elsewhere and the stents are buying just hours or days of hospitalized time. It is easier, and more remunerative, for these specialists to promise a new joint, a new valve, or a stented duct than to discuss the many reasons not to proceed, especially when other physicians carry the burden of hospital care.

The physicians promoting a clinical trial or a medical appliance, in which they have a financial interest, are not likely to give unvarnished advice. Intellectually, they want their trial to succeed. Financially, they want to be rewarded. Combine a clinical trial with a financial inducement, and the result tends to be a study with suspiciously good outcomes that are hard to reproduce.

My perspective on the commercialization of medical care may seem overly harsh. Commercialization of care has driven some technologies and many medical advances. But the application of medical technology should not be indiscriminate, and the elderly should not be treated without appreciation for the limited benefits that they are likely to accrue.

The paradigm shift we need is not a technical one; it is a spiritual, emotional, or intellectual one. We do not need encouragement to believe in miracles. We need to understand that there will not be an endless series of miracles. We need to stop believing that advances that are likely to help young people will equally benefit old people. When old age is a diagnosis, treatments are a zero-sum game. Fixing one system puts further strain on the others. "Buying some time" means getting one more day of hospitalization and side effects at the expense of losing a day at home in comparative comfort.

AN ANALYSIS OF A GOOD DEATH

Karen Kehl concludes that the attributes of a good death are (in order of decreasing importance) being in control, being comfortable, having a sense of closure, being valued as a person, trusting one's care providers, recognizing the impending death, honoring beliefs, minimizing the burden, optimizing relationships, utilizing the appropriate amount of technology, leaving a legacy, and being cared for by family.[2]

Of these twelve attributes, most require advance planning. Although, according to the study, recognizing the impending death is the seventh most important attribute, without that recognition, one cannot plan and without planning one cannot be in control, have a sense of closure, enjoy being valued as a person, have one's beliefs honored, or optimize relationships.

To me, these are emotional attributes of a good death. Equally important are the physical attributes of a comfortable death, utilizing the appropriate amount of technology and being cared for by family. These, too, require advance planning and a vision. The eighth attribute, minimizing the burden, could be an emotional or financial judgment into which I will not wade. The eleventh attribute, leaving a legacy, requires planning, but is a lifetime achievement attribute, not an end-of-life proposition.

Given that nine of the twelve attributes of a good death require enough advance planning to achieve control, comfort, closure, self-worth, trust, honored beliefs, the setting of choice, and family care, I maintain that understanding and acknowledging illness, in concert with a vision of the end, is central to achieving a better death.

If we accept the preceding as the attributes of a good death, then the attributes of a bad death are losing control (not in accord with wishes, not in location of choice, prolonged, dependent, traumatic), suffering (in pain or distress, cognitively impaired, fearful, or angry), being unprepared, being subjected to disorganized care, lacking knowledge of impending death, being a burden to the family, being alone, and being young. Except for the final condition, the remaining attributes of a bad death define a medicalized death in the ICU or a warehoused death in an institution.

HOW YOU CAN TAKE CONTROL: SPECIFIC STEPS

If you are reading this book, you are forward thinking. You may be an aging patient. You may be the caregiver (or potential caregiver) for an aging patient. You might be someone reflecting on the recent death experience of a family member or acquaintance and wondering how to do it better. In any event, most readers will think that the ideas outlined here are not really for them, at least not right now. I agree.

If you live independently, drove to the store, bought this book, and are reading it unaided, you probably do not think of yourself as a candidate to institute any of the concrete steps I describe, except to have a firmly written advance directive. If you have such an advance directive you might think that your job is done. It is not. If you want to increase the likelihood of a better death, you have much more work to do.

For those who are lucky enough to reach an advanced age, that age must become part of medical decision making.

Adjust your life style to emphasize safety. Be responsible about facing your physical shortcomings and avoiding unsafe terrain. We protect toddlers from unsafe terrain. Take precautions. Protect yourself from falls. Embrace a cane or walker. Avoid unsafe activities.

Review your family network. Do you have the option, means, and resources to die at home? Look into the burgeoning options for health care and assistance at home. There is an explosion of businesses and social service agencies supplying domestic services, home health aides, and nursing services to help the elderly "age in place." Review them.

Consider assisted living and nursing home options. Review the nursing home policy on natural death and self-dehydration. Find one consistent with your views. Review the opinions of the nursing home medical director. Find one consistent with your views.

Review your advance care planning. Discuss this with your agent, relatives, and close friends. Establish a series of agents, recognizing that at a critical moment your primary agent might be unavailable.

Study your jurisdictional options for end-of-life decisions. Most states have, or are developing, an expanded set of Do Not Resuscitate–type orders that address treatment decisions common to seriously ill or frail patients. These are known as POLST (Physician Orders for Life-Sustaining Treatment) or MOLST (Medical Orders for Life-Sustaining Treatment) orders, and they are explained in Appendix I on Advance Directives. How does your jurisdiction treat the presence of a Do Not Resuscitate bracelet? Does your state have a mature POLST program? Does your state have right-to-die laws?

Choose an age to start the process of conservative decision making. Assert your understanding that medical intervention in the aged is a blunted instrument with diminished benefits. Ezekiel Emanuel has chosen age seventy-five. This is intentionally provocative and arbitrarily premature. But it makes the point that age-related decisions must be made. So choose an age to start the process of rethinking aggressive treatments and low-yield screening exams. If you reach eighty to ninety years of age without a chronic illness, or seventy to eighty years of age with one of the major chronic illnesses, take stock of your situation. Consider rejecting non-palliative medical intervention.

Consult a geriatrician. Discuss your illnesses and condition. Discuss your medications. Discuss your prognosis. Discuss the limits of screening and prevention. Discuss sensible, age-appropriate decision making. If you are at the average life expectancy for your demographic or if you have a chronic illness and your primary care physician insists on continued screening mammography, screening colonoscopy, screening chest X-rays, EKGs, screening urinalysis, inter alia, they are probably exaggerating the benefits of these tests and are not working with your best interests in mind. Transfer your care to the geriatrician.

Review your clinical diagnosis. Develop a vision of your death. Where do you want to die—at home, in a hospital, in a nursing home? Can you see how death might come—from pneumonia, dehydration, or a heart attack? When the time comes, can you influence the timing of your death by refusing treatments, medication, or fluid and food?

Study your prognosis. What is the course of your chronic illness? What is your personal trajectory? Can you see when death might come? Can you build an exit strategy around that? What exit options can you foresee? Build them into your advance directive.

Study your performance status. Do you have less energy? Do you need household help? Recognize that the progressive acquisition of household help means a reduction in performance status is occurring.

Study the trajectory of your performance status. If, as a result of age or disease, you have noticed increasing limitations on your daily activities with difficulty bathing or toileting, transferring from bed to chair, or if you need help eating, discuss a passive approach to medical care.

Study your disease trajectory. Do you recognize a cyclical pattern of harsher treatments and less successful rehabilitation? Are your doctors locked in a "test and treat" mode? If you have been hospitalized four times in the last year, if you have had multiple courses of chemotherapy, if you have had several emergency room visits for fall-related trauma, if you have any chronic symptoms that are not being well managed, then seek a palliative care consultation.

Discuss DNR and POLST orders with your physician. If you are elderly and frail, CPR is extremely unsuccessful. The same is true if you are over sixty-five and have a chronic illness. Strongly consider a DNR status.[3] If available in your state, discuss POLST orders with your physician, and do so well in advance of the time to execute them. They are designed to complement the living will. Therefore, coordinate and reconcile these two documents. If not coordinated, the more recently executed document takes precedence.

Consider hospice care early in the course of a terminal diagnosis. Study the attitudes and quality measures of local hospices. If you have the means to pay for hospice care, seek out a hospice that has good-quality metrics and will consider admission prior to federal government eligibility requirements. If you do not have the means for private pay hospice care, seek admission as early as possible based on a generous and loose interpretation of the federal guidelines. Hospices have the services to prevent unnecessary ER visits, overdiagnosis, and overtreatment. Later in the hospice course, consider your medication list. Delete the medications designed to prolong life. Delete the medications with any unpleasant side effects. Continue the medications that promote comfort and well-being. Understand the medications that have the potential to induce a coma or an arrhythmia. When the time comes, institute your exit strategy.

Review all decisions with your agent and your family. Share your vision with your family. Rehearse scenarios. Keep in mind, as you read this now, you are of sound mind and sound enough body. However, at some point in the future you will not be so sound. It is very likely that you will engage in a consultation with an ER doctor or an ICU physician. Under those circumstances you might meet the technical definition of mental competence, but disease, medication, and fatigue will have clouded your thinking. Then you will need and want an agent to stand by you and to engage the physician in a way that best represents your current and former wishes.

Interweaving the education of your agents about your advance directive with a geriatric consultation, age-related medical decision making, early DNR status, plans for POLST orders, early hospice admission, and an appreciation for a natural death is the formula that minimizes the likelihood of suffering painful, futile treatments.

YOU ARE NOT GIVING UP

It may be too early to institute the final stages, but it is never too early for an adult to start this planning. If you are reading this and feeling perplexed, the time is not right to take the advance steps. When the time is right, you will know it.

When a patient accepts their illness or debility, they are not giving up. When a patient understands the course of their illness, they are able to plan. When a patient dictates therapy, be it passive or aggressive, they are taking control. But when a patient chooses open-ended treatment they are placing some, or all, control into the hands of others.

Treating doctors treat. Surgeons operate. Internists prescribe.

Nephrologists dialyze. Pulmonologists ventilate. Cardiologists implant pacemakers and defibrillators. Gastroenterologists scope and stent narrowed orifices. Oncologists administer chemotherapy. Interventional radiologists open narrowed blood vessels and stent weakened blood vessels. All of these treatments have a time and place, but their role at an advanced age or near the end of life should be reviewed, analyzed, questioned, and minimized.

All of these treatments, before the end of life, are justifiable. Toward the end of life when dealing with a terminal illness, before the illness segues into a terminal condition, they might be justifiable. But at some point, a combination of age, diminished performance status, and disease render these treatments inappropriate. At that point, these treatments "buy some time," at best, or cause a complication and "lose some time," at worst. There are no easy answers. There are no absolutely right or absolutely wrong answers, but do not be blinded by false hope.

MY MOTHER'S UROSEPSIS

My mother suffered from an episode of urosepsis a few months before she died. That episode illustrates several points about the importance of sharing her vision, having a strong and informed agent to stand up for her, and that being in hospice was not synonymous with "giving up."

One month before my daughter's wedding, I was visiting my parents. One morning my mother woke up in a confused state. At my direction, she was admitted to the hospital for the "disorientation" of sepsis. She was not in pain. The admitting physician, new to her case, remembered that she did not want to be aggressive but he had forgotten about her goal of surviving to see her granddaughter get married.

He did not order IV antibiotics "because she was a DNR and enrolled in home hospice care." This was a gross misinterpretation of our acceptance of her terminal lung cancer diagnosis. We had not yet discussed with him the possibility of using sepsis as an exit opportunity. We would not have brought her to the hospital if we wanted to decline antibiotics at that point. A Do Not Resuscitate/hospice status is not equivalent to a comfort-care-only status—that comes later. Some treatments are justifiable, such as antibiotics, when there is a clear goal in mind. My mother, sleepy from her illness, could not speak for herself. And my father, confused by the crush of events, did not notice the absence of the antibiotics. Fortunately, after I took the admitting MD to task, they were started in time to bring her around. Her vision was to die at home after the wedding. She did not want to give up to this particular infection. And I, knowing her plans, was able to speak up for her.

ACCEPTING DEATH DOES NOT MEAN WANTING TO DIE

Until the very end of their lives, my parents were not depressed, nor did they want to die. My parents never asked for an easy way out. They did not seek a miraculous cure. They did not ask for a suicide pill.

But my parents did not want to suffer. They did not want to live in a state of decline and decrepitude. My mother avoided that by acknowledging her terminal diagnosis. My father enjoyed three good years after strengthening his aneurysm. But by eliminating that exit strategy, he paid the price with two years of decline, and he did slip into decrepitude. Wisely, he minimized its duration by refusing further medical treatment, entering hospice, and discontinuing his routine medications.

They knew that death was inevitable. They knew this not simply as an intellectual proposition. They knew it in their hearts. They knew, instinctively, that fighting for life was the way to medicalize their death and to make the process crueler than it had to be. They knew that planning for death was the way to gain a modicum of control and to maintain a modicum of dignity.

To accept that death is inevitable is the first step toward peace. To be ready to die at the appropriate time is the foundation for a better death. Neither readiness nor acceptance indicates that one wants to die—although, when suffering develops, a desire to hasten death might also develop. This happened to my father when, during the last months of his life, his dependence on others contributed to an existential pain and his decision to discontinue non-palliative medications.

I do not know why my parents were so sensible. I do not know why they were ready to die when death came to them. Had I taught them a little with my stories of training and practice? Possibly, but I don't think so. Had they taught me about their perspective on death with their visits to ailing friends and neighbors? Certainly.

They knew that death was about dying, not fighting futilely to live progressively diminished lives.

They knew that the important things at the end of life are not the acts of fighting the dying process, but engaging in the living process.

Abridged Chronology:
Mom and Dad's Decline

IN 2007, MY PARENTS were a comparatively healthy elderly couple. My mother was nearing eighty-two. My father was closing in on eighty-six. They lived quietly in a spacious apartment in a frayed-at-the-edges second-rate residential hotel overlooking downtown Milwaukee and the western shore of Lake Michigan.

My father was robust for his age, a condition that he had not earned in his youth either by exercising physically or by exercising restraint.

My mother was frail. She had suffered multiple osteoporosis-related fractures over the years. She had minimal exercise tolerance. Trips through the airport required the aid of a wheelchair. She was slightly demented. Her conversations were punctuated with gambits to cover forgotten facts. She was generally sedentary but was surprisingly motivated by hair appointments, shopping trips, and family visits.

In January of 2007, while visiting their second daughter in California, she developed a cough, subsequently diagnosed as pneumonia. As is frequently the case, resolution of the pneumonia revealed an underlying lung cancer. She entered home hospice care in March. She was hospitalized for a kidney infection in April. She attended my daughter's wedding in May. She died quietly, at home, in September 2007.

My father soldiered on. He stayed in their apartment. He traveled alone, re-creating their annual trips to each of their children. In the winter he returned to California, where their second daughter and her large stepfamily hosted him. He followed that with his regular trip to Florida, where his eldest daughter hosted him. In the spring he visited me in Washington and his youngest daughter in Virginia. During the summer he flew to Down East Maine, no small feat for an octogenarian. He made two solo trips to Europe, attended multiple family events and multiple descendants' graduations.

In 2009, he had an outpatient procedure to strengthen his abdominal aortic aneurysm. In the spring of 2010, he met his first great-grandchild.

At that point, age was creeping up on him. He hired some college students to act as attendants to help him with routine daily chores. We hired an outpatient nursing service to monitor his health, distribute his medications, and accompany him to doctor visits.

Between 2010 and 2013, he curtailed his travel. He made his last trip to Maine in 2011 at age ninety, wearing diapers (just in case), using a wheelchair in the airport, and using a cane. He made his last trips to Florida and California in late 2012 and early 2013. By this time he needed a travel companion, and my sisters divided this duty.

Between 2013 and 2014, he curtailed his social activities. He dined out only with visiting family members. He used a walker for short walks and a transfer chair for longer distances. His young attendants were helping him get up in the morning and go to bed at night. Once a week, a woman, hired through the nursing service, came in to prepare a fresh meal to be served hot to my father and one or two dinner guests. She also prepared six meals to be refrigerated or frozen and to be microwaved and served by his young assistants.

In August of 2014, three minor falls near his bedside prompted a shift to twenty-four-hour coverage by attendants hired through the nursing service. In September, he began to use a wheelchair to move around the apartment. In October, he was accepted into a hospice program.

In December of 2014, Dad decided to refuse his routine medications. By January of 2015, he required complete assistance to transfer from bed to chair. His last trip to the opera was in March. By April he needed two people and a mechanical lift to transfer him from bed to chair. On April 14, he refused the mechanical lift and he took to bed. On April 21, he stopped eating and drinking. On April 25, 2015, he died quietly.

APPENDIXES

Appendix I

Advance Directives

Why would I want to fix something that is going to carry me away the way that I want to go?
—John T. Harrington, during a conversation with the author

―――――――

Why is advance care planning so important? Because without it you have ceded control of your end-of-life care to medical professionals dedicated to treatment at all cost. Under these circumstances you are likely to undergo futile treatment that is painful and that isolates you from your friends and family.

Even though any verbal guidance you give your family and friends is likely to play the largest role in the implementation of your advance care planning, for purposes of this chapter, I focus on the written documents and their special roles in end-of-life care. This is an impossibly dry subject, so let's cut to the chase.

There are three roles for the written documents involved in advance care planning. The first is to remind your agent of your wishes as translated from conversations into the written word through the very act of creating the content of these documents. The second is to instruct your physicians in exactly what care to implement when the directives are written as medical orders (a Do Not Resuscitate order, for example). And the third is to inform a judge in the unlikely and unfortunate event of a legal battle.

Now let's get right to some simplified definitions.

ADVANCE DIRECTIVES: DEFINITIONS

The legalities of the process have created multiple terms that get bandied about such as Living Will, Proxy Directive, Personal Directive, Health Care Proxy, Agent, Durable Power of Attorney for Health Care, Do Not Resuscitate orders, Physician Orders for Life-Sustaining Treatment (POLST), and others. There are many jurisdictional variations in terminology and statutes guiding care.[1] For purposes of this chapter, an advance directive is any written or verbal request that expresses an end-of-life wish as part of advance care planning. The "Advance Directive" is the nearly universal term applied to a specific document that combines a "living will" and a "durable power of attorney for health care"—the patient's representative.

For purposes of this chapter, I will offer the following definitions with the goal of supplying simple, understandable, and acceptable "umbrella" terminology.

Definitions of Advance Care Planning Terminology

Advance Directive: A document combining the potentially separate legal documents of a living will and a durable power of attorney for health care.

Living Will: The subsection of the Advance Directive that addresses the patient's desires, goals, ideas and, ultimately, their end-of-life wishes.

Durable Power of Attorney for Health Care: The subsection of the Advance Directive that gives health care decision-making power to a person (proxy or agent) on behalf of the patient (grantor). It is "durable" because the power endures even when the grantor is incapacitated.

Agent: The person (or persons) named to act on behalf of the patient in the durable power of attorney for health care.

Do Not Resuscitate: Physician orders that are most commonly used in a patient's hospital chart indicating that in the event of cardiorespiratory arrest no electric shock, chest compressions, or artificial ventilation is to be applied in an attempt to restart the heart or stimulate breathing. DNR is synonymous with "No CPR" (No Cardio-Pulmonary Resuscitation) or "No Code." The acronym DNR is being replaced in some hospitals by AND, which means "allow natural death."

DNR orders can also exist as a transportable legal form outside the hospital. In this case they are signed by a physician and establish that the patient has chosen a legal status that is to be honored anywhere within their jurisdiction by providers (doctors, nurses, paramedics, and emergency medical technicians) in the event of unexpected cardiac arrest. This document is usually accompanied by a bracelet or necklace worn by the patient and registered with the state. DNR orders are a form of advance directive but in most jurisdictions they exist separately from the living will.

POLST (Physician Orders for Life-Sustaining Treatment): A transportable set of physician orders that document a conversation between a patient and his or her primary care physician. In the event of an emergency, they order a plan of action for first responders, ER physicians, attending physicians, and nursing home staff.

Like an expanded DNR order, POLST orders address treatment decisions common to seriously ill or frail patients and include guidance about comfort measures, nutritional support, and antibiotics. POLST orders standardize the patient's wishes in the form of doctor's orders in a portable plan of care. The orders are printed on eye-catching pink or green paper that is to be kept on the patient's refrigerator door or the nursing home bed. They are to be transported to the hospital or emergency room with the patient. If they are overlooked by emergency personnel and do not arrive at the hospital with the patient, their value is lost.

POLST orders are not available in many jurisdictions. Although most states are developing POLST programs, such programs are well established in only a minority of states. In those states where POLST programs are mature, all emergency personnel look for and all physicians promote and respect such orders. Where programs are not well established, these orders might be overlooked or ignored.

It is critical to note the difference between the wishes outlined in a living will and the orders documented in the DNR and POLST forms. In a clinical setting, the "wishes" require interpretation by the treating physician but the "orders"—having been signed by the primary care physician—are to be followed by the treating physician without question or reinterpretation. The importance of this distinction will become clearer with subsequent examples.

How These Documents Interact and Overlap

The Durable Power of Attorney

During the creation of an Advance Directive, most forms will first require the patient to fill out the durable power of attorney for health care. This is simply the form that identifies the agent (or, better yet, a series of agents) who will act on behalf of the patient. It is understood that the agent will act when the patient is incompetent. But agents can also act on the patient's behalf (make appointments, schedule tests, receive information) at any time the patient is tired or sick.

The agent is usually a relative (spouse, sibling, child) or close friend, but they can be a primary care physician or lawyer.[2]

Keep in mind that during consultations with physicians, most families work as a de facto committee with the agent serving as the chairman or the ultimate arbiter. Some family members might not agree with the treatment wishes outlined in the living will. If they tend to be disruptive, you (the patient or agent) should consider excluding such individuals from participating in those discussions either as a stipulation of the Advance Directive or as an ad hoc instruction at the time of an important clinical decision. Excluding family members, though occasionally necessary, is bound to create friction, so give it careful thought and try to avoid it.

The Living Will

The living will, as a subset of the Advance Directive, outlines end-of-life wishes. These can be very broad or very detailed. For example, where I currently reside, the state-supplied boilerplate is very broad and the form requests that patients check a box:

☐ Choice not to be kept alive:

  I do not want treatment to keep me alive if my physician decides that either of the following is true;

  i) I have an illness that will not get better, cannot be cured, and will result in my death quite soon (sometimes referred to as a terminal condition), or

  ii) I am no longer aware (unconscious) and it is very likely that I will never be conscious again (sometimes referred to as a persistent vegetative state).

☐ Choice to be kept alive

  I want to be kept alive as long as possible within the limits of generally acceptable health care standards, even if my condition is terminal or I am in a persistent vegetative state.

Please note, there are a few more detailed questions later in this state's advance directive form and there are blank areas for the author to add a few personalized thoughts or wishes. But not all questions have to be answered, and checking one of these two boxes creates a legally adequate document.

More important, note the degree of interpretation required of the emergency room physician when presented with this document and an unattended (no agent is yet present) nursing home patient who is near death—semi-conscious, with low blood pressure, and a weak heart rhythm. Even if the first box is checked, because the doctor does not know the underlying diagnosis (in this example, it is likely to be sepsis, but it could be something even less treatable) and does not know the patient's recent mind-set about aggressive therapy, they are likely to proceed with aggressive diagnosis and treatment. Given the circumstances described, it is appropriate that they do so. POLST orders, described on page 235, would have altered this dynamic.

Do Not Resuscitate

The next level of advance directive is the Do Not Resuscitate (DNR) form. In most jurisdictions, a DNR order is a separate document from the Advance Directive. A DNR order is also independent of and can predate POLST orders and hospice status. If so inclined, a patient can obtain a DNR status from their physician long before they can be accepted into a hospice program.

It is appropriate for any patient of advanced years to consider DNR status, even if they are still living independently, because cardiopulmonary resuscitation—contrary to popular belief and media representation—is so traumatic and ineffective, with a success rate of less than 8 percent among the old and frail.[3]

But having a DNR bracelet does not guarantee that resuscitation will not be attempted. When presented with an unknown and otherwise healthy-appearing patient who has just suffered an unexplained cardio-respiratory arrest, some health care workers will overlook or ignore a DNR bracelet or pendant and initiate attempts at resuscitation. POLST orders and hospice care status are more likely to be honored under such duress.

POLST Orders

POLST orders are an attempt to convert the wishes expressed in a living will into doctor's orders to be honored in an emergency situation. These orders address sophisticated end-of-life treatment choices for patients who are frail or chronically ill and who have discussed with their primary care physician those aggressive procedures that they will, or will not, accept in the event of serious illness. Choices to accept or decline cardiopulmonary resuscitation, various levels of breathing support including mechanical ventilation, hemodialysis, antibiotics, transfusions, artificial nutrition, and artificial hydration are variably included in the POLST programs of different states. Because the decisions to accept or reject various treatments are written as pre-existing orders by the primary care physician, emergency personnel and critical care physicians are expected to honor them.

An example of the appropriate use of POLST orders could be as follows. Imagine an eighty-five-year-old woman living semi-independently in an assisted living facility. Having watched her husband die slowly in the associated nursing home, she wants to avoid that fate. If she were to have a large stroke and was taken to the local emergency room with POLST orders stipulating no CPR, no mechanical ventilation, no tube feeding, and no artificial hydration, she would avoid aggressive treatments and be placed in hospice care.

AN EXAMPLE OF A LIVING WILL

"My agent should be guided by the general principle that I do not fear death itself as much as the indignities of deterioration, dependence, and hopeless pain. For example, if I am in the process of dying from an incurable injury or illness from which there is no reasonable possibility of a cure or significant recovery, or if I am in a comatose or persistently vegetative state from which any meaningful recovery of cognitive brain function is highly unlikely, or even if I suffer a combination of nonterminal illnesses which significantly reduces the quality of my life (e.g., Parkinson's disease causing me to choke on my food, osteoporosis giving me severe bone pain, and/or a stroke that has diminished my capacity to communicate), I request that my agent refuse or discontinue my medical treatment which will only prolong the process of my dying or the duration of my irreversible coma or persistent vegetative state.

In those circumstances I do not want cardiac resuscitation, mechanical respiration, dialysis, antibiotics, intravenous alimentation or hydration, tube feeding, or feeding by spoon, glass or straw held by another person if this is likely to be my only mode of alimentation for the foreseeable future.

I believe that the voluntary refusal of enteral alimentation (food) and hydration (fluid) is a comfortable and ethical means to hasten death. I further commend to my agent and to the health care professionals involved in my care the articles in the *New England Journal of Medicine*,

Vol. 349, July 24, 2003, No. 4, at pages 325–326 and 359–65 as further guidance on my views regarding the matters addressed in this paragraph.[4]

I further believe that the combination of two or more non-terminal illnesses may diminish the quality of my life sufficiently to warrant hastening the inevitability of death by voluntary dehydration, and if I am unable to communicate effectively, I direct my agent to refuse or discontinue such medical treatment on my behalf.

I do, however, want maximum pain relief even though pain relief drugs or procedures may lead to permanent damage or addiction or may hasten the moment of my death.

These examples should not be interpreted as limitations of the general principle stated in this paragraph. In addition, I direct that my agent make decisions consistent with any other principles, instructions and desires that I may have stated to my agent or to others orally or in writing. In the absence of such statements, my agent may make the decisions for me that my agent believes to be in my best interests."

These paragraphs are taken from my parents' living wills and are a good example of spelling out clearly the issues of prolonging the process of dying, manual feeding, self-dehydration, and adequate pain medication—common stumbling blocks in end-of-life care.

If offered an opportunity to update it, I would probably make several changes.

First, I would add a more specific dementia clause[5] and a transfer clause.[6] Second, I would probably make use of the term "exit option" or "exit strategy." There my intent would be to let my agent and the reader know that I think invoking such a strategy is appropriate. Third, I would elaborate on the use of antibiotics and would add that a septic death, accompanied by pain and anxiety medications, might be a specific goal, a specific exit option. As indicated in chapter 5, a septic death is usually quick and comparatively comfortable. I might add a specific clause to the document, and give verbal instructions to my agents, that sepsis should be considered as the cause of any altered mental status, and treatment of sepsis should be specifically avoided.

CREATING YOUR OWN ADVANCE DIRECTIVE

The goal of an Advance Directive is to outline the principles of care to be rendered at end of life. The goal of this appendix is to help the reader comfortably develop the most effective Advance Directive that will suit your needs.

You do not need a lawyer or doctor to draft a legally binding and medically adequate Advance Directive. Filling out your state's boilerplate form will suffice if properly witnessed and notarized when required. But if you want to add clarifying detail for a more comprehensive and binding document, you will want professional help to avoid contradictions, maintain legal compliance, and to better understand the medical implications of your choices.

For researching discussion points, there are multiple organizations that have advice to offer. Two such organizations, **Caring Connections** (a program of the National Hospice and Palliative Care Organization) and **Compassion & Choices** (formerly The Hemlock Society and currently promoting medical aid in dying) have websites that deal extensively with end-of-life issues. Either of their associated websites (**caringinfo.org** or **compassionandchoices.org**) can guide you to your state's suggested Advance Directive or help you create one of your own.

Because Compassion & Choices does promote medical aid in dying (formerly "physician assisted suicide" or "death with dignity"), its website is replete with provocative information and it presents hypothetical scenarios designed to stimulate your thoughts on these and other subjects.

From the perspective of keeping it simple, **Aging With Dignity** (**agingwithdignity.org**) is a nonprofit organization dedicated to promoting human dignity during the aging and dying process. They offer an easy to use, less medically oriented, Advance Directive called Five Wishes. Written in plain language and touching on spiritual and emotional aspects of the dying process, Five Wishes is a comprehensive document that serves to satisfy the requirements of an Advance Directive in forty-two states. Its simple language is particularly good at creating the verbal communication that is so important to fleshing out the written word. Even if you have another Advance Directive, you can use Five Wishes as a tool to work through most of the important questions your family should be asking about end-of-life issues.

Finally, once drafted, you should review your Advance Directive with your agent, your family, and your primary care physician— particularly if they did not play a role in its creation. As many people as possible should be in the know and in agreement.

PARSING FULL CARE: A TRIAL OF LIMITED CARE VERSUS PALLIATION

An interesting idea forwarded in some advance directives includes the concept of trying to compromise between aggressive treatment and palliative care. This usually takes the form of a trial period for certain therapies—hoping that recovery will be better than predicted. A trial of tube feeding for several weeks following a massive stroke is one such example.

This is also a common discussion point at end-of-life bedside con-sultations for the inadequately prepared agent and family trying to work out a compromise with the attending cardiologist or the ICU physician. Grandma is dying but they just can't let go, so instead of saying no to antibiotics for a serious pneumonia, they say, "Please don't put her on the breathing machine again, but try antibiotics for three days and if she is no better then we can stop them."

In my clinical experience, these compromise scenarios never worked out well. They always prolong the decision making, which means more suffering for the patient, and because they are compro-mises they never allow the use of every resource, essentially guarantee-ing failure. I do not see how institutionalizing a trial period can help where a yes or no answer is that which is truly needed. Medicine at the very end of life should be full bore or full stop.

THE OTHER PERSPECTIVE ON END-OF-LIFE WISHES: TRYING TO LIVE FOREVER

It is quite possible that my concepts of aggressive passivity and exit strategies do not appeal to you. Then you should make that clear in your Advance Directive. If you want to aggressively treat every acute and chronic illness despite progressive incapacity, dependence on mechanical support, and the development of a persistent vegetative state, those specific instructions should be included in your living will, as a kindness to your family.

It is the minority of families where all members hold the same principles of end-of-life care. Some families have members who think that patients should fight on, forever, and against all odds. In the same family, there may be others who encourage accepting what fate has come to offer. Those latter family members will be very uncomfortable watching you survive in a persistent vegetative state or struggle for an extended time on a ventilator. Only by firmly stipulating—verbally and in writing—that it is your wish "to be kept alive for as long as possible within the limits of generally accepted health care standards" will you keep them from trying to influence the process.

With this perspective in mind, you might want to include a paragraph on your religious beliefs and the possibility of miracles or your confidence in scientific progress to address all problems.

You might also want to include a transfer clause asking to be moved from a facility pressuring your family to discontinue life support to a facility (should one be available) willing to continue it.

THE TIMING OF WRITTEN DIRECTIVES

Here is a reminder as to how these documents should be created in sequence and the appropriate timing for their creation.

Every adult member of society should have an Advance Directive. Young adults, at a minimum, should address the desire (or lack thereof) to be kept alive in the event of a terminal illness or vegetative state and the treatment choices to be considered (CPR, mechanical ventilation, hemodialysis, artificial nutrition or artificial hydration, among others) or declined. At this point an agent should be identified if it might be someone other than a parent or spouse.

As a person ages the Advance Directive should be refined. A sequence of agents should be established. Details to address multiple death scenarios should be added. Such refinements should also acknowledge new diagnoses and the death scenarios associated with each applicable chronic illness.

If an accumulation of age and illness make a five-year survival unlikely, a patient might seek a DNR status in addition to strengthening their Advance Directive.

If a patient and doctor recognize that circumstances predict a one- or two-year survival, then POLST orders are appropriate and should be targeted to the specific diseases involved.

Finally, when a six- to twelve-month survival is postulated, hospice care should be introduced. At this point, the Advance Directive, DNR order, and POLST orders are folded into the hospice philosophy and day-to-day decisions are made based on the latter but reinforced by the former.

ORAL VERSUS WRITTEN DIRECTIVES

The most important thing to remember about Advance Directives is that the written word serves as a communication tool to the agent and the family and an outline for the authorities as to the intent and the wishes of the patient. The written word is uncommonly invoked and rarely parsed closely when a doctor has to make critical care decisions.

Most decisions at the-end-of-life are made in real time, in the form of verbal communication between the patient, doctor, agent, and family. Therefore, reviewing the contents of the living will and rehearsing the concepts of your advance care planning are critically important. As long as the patient remains competent, their verbal instructions define the agenda for any clinical situation. When the patient is borderline competent, as is frequently the case, or incompetent, a unified family that is led by an informed agent will dictate the direction of care. Physicians will not ask to see the living will in such circumstances.

However, under the pressure of emergency care, and facing a divided family, a physician is more likely to defy the actual agent who says, "No treatment," while two agitated siblings are saying, "Yes, do everything." In this case the patient will be exposed to unwanted and painful treatment until the living will can be reviewed.

Only in the most extraordinary circumstances does the Advance Directive get closely parsed. Most of them would involve a legal scenario in which two entities (the hospital and the patient's family, for example) have competing interests and the patient is not competent to express himself or herself. It is at that point that the legal drafting is most important and the examples of extra clauses and clinical scenarios become most critical.

ADVANCE DIRECTIVE AND EXIT STRATEGY

A patient's Advance Directive should be formulated with their wishes, exclusively, in mind. If your goal is to live as long as possible, no matter what the cost or with what quality of life, then there is little need to consider limitations on care. But you should, specifically, state this intent to spare observers the angst of watching the drawn-out process.

If a natural death is the goal, it should be clear in the living will that the quality of life is more important than quantity. It should also be clear that the author of the living will fears the indignities of deterioration, dependence, and hopeless pain more than death itself.

If you want to aim at the "good death," the natural death, described in this book, then your Advance Directive should focus on that. You need to use it as part of an exit strategy.

Things to Remember/Things to Consider

- Your written Advance Directive instructs your agents and informs the legal system of your wishes.
- A shared vision informs your agent and family
- Your verbal directions, or those of your agent, supersede previously written directives.
- At bedside consultations, a unified family will ease decision making; a conflicted family will complicate decision making and possibly contravene the Advance Directive.

Appendix II

Dementia

I want to tell you how much I miss my mother. Bits of her are still there. I miss her most when I am sitting across from her.
—Candy Crowley, CNN correspondent

There are several forms of confusion and memory loss that can be mistaken for dementia. Some of these are treatable and might be reversible.[1] However, there is no effective treatment for true dementia. For this chapter, I am referring to those more common forms of dementia that are relentlessly progressive and fatal. I will use Alzheimer's disease and dementia interchangeably.

Dementia is a special problem for end-of-life care. The unique reversal of mental decline before physical decline raises two questions. The first is how to impose one's will on end-of-life events when one's mastery of one's will and intellect are gone. The second is even more problematic. With respect to every other chronic illness, the lessons of this book are designed to avoid a medicalized death "too late" in life. With Alzheimer's, how can you (via your agent) avoid a death that is too late and yet, not "too early"?

Alzheimer's has one of the most predictable courses of any chronic disease. In the absence of another chronic illness dictating events, it moves through recognizable stages. The early stages include periods of competence and an acceptable quality of life. The later stages are marked by incompetence and social withdrawal before the spiral into debility and a poor, possibly unacceptable, quality of life. The advanced phases may also include personality changes before physical disability sets in. Finally, where dementia is the dominant disease process, and without death by some other acute process, a bed-bound existence—potentially years in duration—awaits, and death will come very late by an infection such as aspiration pneumonia or some other, less predictable, event.

This is because, in general, for any given functional level, a demented patient will live longer than a functionally matched patient with a different chronic disease. In fact, if a patient with cancer, heart failure, or one of the other chronic illnesses suffers a 70 percent decline on the Karnofsky Performance Scale, they qualify for hospice admission. The same decline occurring in a patient suffering exclusively of Alzheimer's disease simply describes them as severely disabled, probably bed-bound, and yet still having a median survival of sixteen months—too long to meet Medicare requirements for hospice admission.

Without a competent patient's input, it is always emotionally harder to forgo treatment. As a result, the agent and family members will be making many medical decisions over many years before any of the final wishes outlined in the advance care planning become appropriate.

MISSION CREEP IN DEMENTIA

By the time a demented patient might have come to the conclusion they had lived too long, and in a competent state would have instructed the doctors and their agent to withhold aggressive medical care, the agent would have established a treatment pattern for them.

For example, during the long period of time that a patient is comparatively physically healthy but modestly cognitively impaired, the agent might have treated a urinary tract infection because the caretakers noted frequent urination and solicited a complaint of cramps or burning. They are likely to have okayed antibiotics for aspiration pneumonia. The agent might have agreed to the use of a blood thinner for the interval development of atrial fibrillation and that in turn required more medical follow-up than originally intended. The agent almost certainly would have treated the trauma of the falls that are guaranteed to occur with dementia and might have done more in terms of treatment and follow-up than a cognitively intact person would allow. It can be very hard to discontinue a pattern of treatment.

My experience is that it is much harder to decline medical treatment on behalf of a fairly hale and hearty patient, even if significantly demented, than it is to withhold treatment from a very frail patient who can still verbalize "no." As a result, between the development of mental incompetence and physical infirmity, multiple medical problems will have occurred, multiple treatments begun, and multiple compromises made. This has the effect of muting the intent of any advance care plans designed to limit medical care.

By the time a demented patient is unable to swallow food or sip liquids they are likely to have been bedridden for a long time. They might have been unable to recognize or relate to friends and family for years. They might have had significant personality changes. They certainly would have been incompetent and unable to reaffirm their intentions as outlined in their advance care planning. In the final analysis, agents, doctors, and scholars (both medical and legal) struggle with effecting the end-of-life wishes of a demented patient even though the guidance was created when cognitively intact.

This is a moral, ethical, and legal quandary that will not soon go away. But when a physician's dual responsibilities to sustain life and relieve suffering are in conflict, we must let the patient's preferences—as we understand them—prevail. Therefore, if a responsible family chooses a path that is an approximation of the patient's previously stated and written desires and if those desires do not transgress the applicable state laws, most end-of-life providers will respect those decisions.

TREATING ADVANCED DEMENTIA CAUSES SUFFERING

People with advanced dementia are fundamentally changed. They are not their former selves. They have dramatically reduced cognition. They frequently develop a new and different personality. They may not recognize their family. They do not know night from day. They become intellectually incapable of self-care (cooking, feeding, bathing, toileting) while they are still physically able to harm themselves (wandering, falling, ingesting unsafe food and fluid). They frequently do not understand what their caregivers are doing when bathing and dressing them.

Advanced Alzheimer's patients never understand medical interventions and actively resist medical care. In hospitals and nursing homes they pull out IVs, drainage tubes, feeding tubes, and bladder catheters. These behaviors cause them harm.

As dementia progresses, so does a patient's withdrawal from society. As the physical decline of severe dementia progresses patients become bed-bound. In this state, despite the best efforts of nursing home staff, the limbs contract and stiffen, locking patients into mummified positions and making bedsores a constant threat. In the absence of advance directives to the contrary, these patients make cyclical trips to the hospital for antibiotic treatments of urinary infections and pneumonia.

As the medical and nursing staff, not yet jaded to such scenes, struggle to straighten an arm or leg to place an IV, they whisper under their breath, "Please, don't let this happen to me."

The fact that severely demented patients suffer long periods of functional disability ending in the incapacitated bed-bound state that most of us want to avoid makes the case for a more powerful, personalized advance directive. This is why agents acting on behalf of demented patients need to be particularly astute at monitoring decline and keenly aware of interval illnesses.

ADVANCE CARE PLANNING FOR DEMENTIA

The special challenges of dementia might benefit by a more sophisticated advance care plan. In the section about Advance Directives, I have recommended that every living will contain a dementia clause. This would be a general statement that in the event of incapacity from advanced dementia the author of the living will would like the agent to invoke the same limitations on medical care as they wished for the circumstance of a terminal illness and comatose condition or a permanent, vegetative state.

But it is clear that the years-long decline from moderate dementia through severe dementia would be intolerable for some readers.[2] In this case, a progressive advance directive should be considered. A progressive directive means that the wishes change as the disease progresses. Recognizing that 50 percent of moderately demented patients have at least one episode of pneumonia before severe dementia sets in, the simplest example of a progressive directive would be to put in writing your desire to refuse antibiotics for pneumonia or sepsis if moderately demented and your desire to reject manual feeding if severely demented.

Next, think more specifically with functional benchmarks in mind. A more comprehensive example of a progressive dementia clause might be:

If I were to be diagnosed with early dementia, my aspiration is to generate an updated living will to reflect the following:

If I am mildly demented and unable to choose the proper clothes for the season or occasion, I want my agent to establish a DNR status; if I am moderately demented and unable to dress, bathe, or toilet myself without assistance, I want my agent to discontinue routine medications, routine doctor visits, antibiotics for infections, and all life-prolonging interventions; and at the first sign of severe dementia (when I am incontinent of stool, unable to walk alone, have speech limited to a few words a day, or am unable to recognize my immediate family) I want to seek hospice admission at the earliest opportunity and I want my family to place a tray of food in front of me but discontinue manual feeding (unless explicitly requested) and allow a natural decline and death.

If a patient with early dementia, while still competent, defines manual feeding as forced medical care (which they can legally decline in the majority of states); if they define the presentation of food and fluid on a tray (from which they can nourish themselves as desired or within their physical limitations) as basic care; then they can offer their own definition of a natural death as occurring when supplied with food but refusing to be fed.

I recognize that this progressive advance directive remains aspirational and will be met with resistance by some caregivers and many institutions. That is why family involvement and admission to an enlightened hospice are probably essential to the act of abiding by a progressive dementia clause. But without this type of directive there is much less hope of avoiding the prolonged bed-bound existence so many of us dread.

DEMENTIA AND A NATURAL DEATH

Even in this age of increasing availability to aid in dying, there is no guarantee that you can avoid years of bed-bound existence with dementia. Even in states with right-to-die laws the mentally incompetent are excluded from the process. Moreover, the quandaries presented by end-of-life care in severe dementia have resulted in legislation in at least four states that have banned the withdrawal of manual feeding.[3]

But by fortifying your advance care plans as just outlined you can maximize the chance of a natural death. To strengthen your resolve in this regard, it is important to reemphasize some points.

First, people have been dying from the complications of dementia for as long as humans have been able to live long enough to develop it. It is natural to die of dementia.

Second, the Patient Self-Determination Act of 1990 makes it legal to decline, withhold, or withdraw medical treatments.

Third, although it may seem more emotionally difficult to withdraw a treatment that is in place than to refuse to start a new treatment, withdrawing and withholding medical treatment are morally, ethically, and legally equivalent.

Fourth, artificial nutrition and hydration are medical treatments. And, in most states, manual feeding is considered a medical treatment, although in a few states it is considered basic care.

Fifth, the Council on Ethical and Judicial Affairs of the American Medical Association stipulates that it is legal and ethical to withhold or withdraw medical care, including artificial nutrition and hydration, from a patient who is incompetent if the agent believes it to be in the patient's best interests.[4]

Finally, for most people, life with dementia is tolerable, even pleasant, up to a certain point. To die prematurely, even with mild dementia, is a tragedy. But for many, life with severe, advanced dementia appears intolerable. And to die too late in life, when life itself is intolerable, can also be tragic.

The legal aspects of withholding food and fluid from an incompetent patient who established guidelines while cognitively intact to refuse ordinary nutrition and hydration have yet to be worked through in every state. But from a medical perspective, the moral and ethical aspects have been accepted. Therefore, if you are inclined to refuse ordinary food and fluid when severely demented as you would in another vegetative state, then you should put it in your living will and trust that your agents will do their best by you.

"BUYING SOME TIME" VERSUS A NATURAL DEATH

Nowhere is the concept of a natural death more important than in the treatment of dementia. Every other chronic illness creates the appearance of sickness. With those illnesses, as death approaches, it looks natural. Not so for most Alzheimer's patients. Moderate dementia does not look like an illness with visible symptoms of chest pain, shortness of breath, cough, fever, bone pain, dramatic weight loss, or stroke. For years after a demented patient becomes incompetent to the time they advance to a bed-bound state, demented patients look healthy and death looks unnatural. But it is not.

Alzheimer's is as terminal a diagnosis as amyotrophic lateral sclerosis and, in a drawn-out sense, as fatal as a massive heart attack. We must constantly remind ourselves of that. We must remind ourselves that the occasional good day is not a sign of reversal of fortune but simply a brief respite from confusion and despair. Before modern medicine, senile patients died naturally as a result of dementia-related illnesses that we can now reverse such as infections, traumas, and self-inflicted toxins. But the ability to treat pneumonia or sepsis does not require us to do so. For treating infections in advanced dementia is prolonging death just as painfully as "buying some time" with chemotherapy is prolonging death in advanced cancer.

Things to Remember/Things to Consider

- Dementia care promotes mission creep.
- Dementia patients suffer.
- Dementia patients look healthy but have a terminal illness.
- Withholding care and withdrawing care are ethically equivalent.
- Forced feeding can be declined, withheld, or withdrawn in most states.

Acknowledgments

I want to thank my sisters, Betsy Moore, Hannah Graziano, and Jane Coble, for the role they played in creating the foundation for this book. They worked together to create a nearly perfect domestic and caregiving environment.

The four of us coordinated frequent visits. We consulted regularly. We shared, in general, our parents' attitudes, and where we differed in details we cooperated to create a unified front. But because I have told this history through my eyes alone, I am responsible for any inaccuracies related to our parents' story.

I want to thank my wife, Debbie Weil, for her editorial oversight, her developmental insight, and the time and effort she took editing my blog posts—a role that markedly improved my writing skills.

My family has played an important role with this project. My daughter Eliza H. Myers, MD, a neonatologist and artist, created the graphics; my son, Timothy Harrington, inspired me with his lawyerly precision; my daughter Amanda Weil Harrington, MD, provided a surgical perspective; my son-in-law, Minor Myers III, provided passes to the Brooklyn Law School Library, where I spent countless hours of writing and revision; my daughter-in-law, Jessica R. Harrington, was supportive throughout; and my parents-in-law, Denie and Frank Weil, were endlessly encouraging, interested, and inspiring.

I would like to thank my book coach, Deborah Reber; my literary agent and friend, Elizabeth Wales, and her assistant, Neal Swain;

Frederick Courtright, who helped me obtain the necessary licenses and permissions; Mónica Miranda, the graphic designer who converted the graphics into digital images; and the entire team at Hachette Book Group/Grand Central Life & Style—most important, my editor, Karen Murgolo; her assistant, Morgan Hedden; Jeff Holt, production editor; and Linda Duggins, publicist.

Thanks also go to those in my current and former communities who helped mold the content and spread the word of my work. Mary Therese O'Donnell, MD, Richard Davis, and Andrea Mitchell offered helpful feedback and support as early readers; Susan Ostertag, MD, and Elizabeth Zentz, MD, offered critical insight as later readers; Dale Russakoff also served as a reader and connected me with Margaret Shapiro, my editor at the *Washington Post*.

Other supporters and contributors include Catherine Hirsch, Jill Hoy, Alyson Hoggart, Judith Jerome, Katy Rinehart, Sally Richardson, Tom and Mary Kay Ricks, Tremaine Smith, Deborah Demille Wagman, and the Blue Hill Public Library, where I spent many hours of rewriting.

I must also thank my former medical partners, Nicholas Christopher, MD, and Thomas M. Loughney, MD; my former colleagues at Sibley Memorial Hospital; and the thousands of patients whom it was my honor to care for over my thirty-one years of medical practice and who served to inspire me to promote the message in this book.

Finally, my family owes an enormous debt to our father's caregivers. I have taken their names from the notebooks they kept over the last two years of his life:

Caregivers: Helen, Gabi, Meagan, Roger, Gayle, Devin, Ann, Connie, Rhonda, and Jackie.

Nurses: Deb and Kit. Hospice personnel: Holly, Julie, and Laura.

Notes

INTRODUCTION

1. Elizabeth Kübler-Ross, *On Death and Dying: What the Dying Have to Teach Doctors, Nurses, Clergy and Their Own Families,* Reprint Edition (New York: Scribner, 2014).
2. Maine POLST (Physician Orders for Life-Sustaining Treatment) Coalition, info@mainehospicecouncil.org.
3. Walter Isaacson (author of *Steve Jobs*), personal email, June 23, 2015.

CHAPTER ONE: JUDGING THE QUALITY OF DEATH— GOOD DEATH, BAD DEATH, BETTER DEATH?

1. It is common for lung cancer to present as pneumonia. That is because the tumor growth narrows the bronchial tree, making it susceptible to bacterial infection. When the infection leads to a cough or fever, the patient visits the doctor. The first chest X-ray shows the cloudy shadow that is diagnostic of pneumonia. When the cloud of infection has cleared on a follow-up X-ray, the cancer mass becomes visible.
2. Median survival is the length of time it takes for 50 percent of patients to die from a given diagnosis. In this example, the median survival for stage IV lung cancer is ten months. Half of all patients will die within ten months and the other half will die sometime later. Again, with respect to lung cancer, most of those who survive for ten months are likely to die in the next two or three months, but a few will survive much longer, thereby extending the "tail" of the survival curve.
3. This ICU scene could have been precipitated by the progression of any number of chronic illnesses, or it could have followed an acute collapse and subsequent cardiopulmonary resuscitation. As portrayed on TV and in the movies CPR is quick, efficient, and successful. In reality it is brutally traumatic and ineffective. If we define the success rate of CPR as discharge from the hospital, then the overall success rate between comparative studies is 8 to 18 percent. Unfortunately, when studied in the old and infirm, it ranges from 0 to 8 percent.

    William J. Ehlenbach, et al., "Epidemiological Study of In-Hospital Cardiopulmonary Resuscitation in the Elderly," *New England Journal of Medicine* 361 (2009): 22–31.

Christoph H. R. Wiese, et al., "Prehospital Emergency Treatment of Palliative Care Patients with Cardiac Arrest: A Retrospective Investigation," *Supportive Care in Cancer* 18, no. 10 (2010): 1287–92.

4. The average life expectancy in the United States is about seventy-nine years. Women tend to live longer than men; the gap is about five years. The current average life expectancy for men is about seventy-seven years and for women it is eighty-two years. The actual numbers vary demographically, with slightly longer life expectancies among the well educated and the well-to-do and shorter life expectancies among the undereducated and poor.

5. The concept of a "good" death is well analyzed by Karen Kehl, RN, et al., in the paper "Moving toward Peace: An Analysis of the Concept of a Good Death," *American Journal of Hospice and Palliative Care* 23, no. 4 (2006): 277–286. She concluded that the attributes of a good death were (in order of decreasing importance) being in control, being comfortable, having a sense of closure, being valued as a person, trusting one's care providers, recognizing the impending death, honoring beliefs, minimizing the burden, optimizing relationships, utilizing the appropriate amount of technology, leaving a legacy, and being cared for by family.

CHAPTER TWO: HOW THE AMERICAN HEALTH CARE SYSTEM FAILS THE ELDERLY

1. From the National Health Expenditure Accounts at CMS.gov, December 6, 2016.

2. The medical-industrial complex and its effects on medical research and clinical decision making prompted the editors of the two most prestigious medical journals to make the following statements:

    "It is simply no longer possible to believe much of the clinical research that is published, or to rely on the judgment of trusted physicians or authoritative medical guidelines. I take no pleasure in this conclusion, which I reached slowly and reluctantly over my two decades as an editor of the *New England Journal of Medicine*." —Marcia Angell, MD, former editor in chief, *New England Journal of Medicine*, 2015.

    "Much of the scientific literature, perhaps half, may simply be untrue. Afflicted by studies with small sample sizes, tiny effects, invalid exploratory analyses, and flagrant conflicts of interest, together with an obsession for pursuing fashionable trends of dubious importance, science has taken a turn towards darkness." —Richard Horton, editor in chief, *The Lancet*, 2015.

3. Hospitalists are physicians hired by a hospital or health care system who work exclusively in the hospital. They have generally come to replace the primary care physicians when a patient is hospitalized. Hospitalists specialize in inpatient problems, the emergency care involved with transferring patients from the ER to the floor and the floor to the ICU, and are particularly familiar with a hospital's electronic medical record and its admission and discharge procedures, thereby making patient care more efficient.

4. H. Gilbert Welch, MD, has written an excellent summary of American medicine's tendency to deliver excessive care in *Overdiagnosed; Making People Sick in*

the Pursuit of Health (Boston: Beacon Press, 2011). He is an expert in the risks and benefits of screening for diseases as part of a preventive medicine strategy.

5. The American Gastroenterology Association, the American Society for Gastrointestinal Endoscopy, the American College of Gastroenterology, the US Preventative Services Task Force, and the American Cancer Society, among others, issue recommendations for colon cancer screening and prevention. These recommendations vary with respect to the emphasis on different tests and the interval between tests. Ongoing research by academic institutions, funded by profit-making companies, regularly questions the validity of these recommendations.

6. The overuse of antibiotics has led to two types of epidemics. One is the rise of bacteria resistant to antibiotics such as the methicillin resistant *Staph. aureus* and the other is the overgrowth of otherwise innocuous organisms such as yeasts or, in this case, *Clostridia difficile.*

7. Sharon Kaufman, *Ordinary Medicine; Extraordinary Treatments, Longer Lives, and Where to Draw the Line* (Durham and London: Duke University Press, 2015).

8. The left ventricular assist device is a battery-powered pumping machine, part of which is worn externally and part of which is inserted into a patient's heart and major blood vessels. It increases the flow of blood from the heart's most important pumping chamber. It was developed as a "bridging" device, to be used in the most advanced cases of heart failure, when the goal is to keep a patient alive in preparation for a potential heart transplant. For many patients, when donor hearts are not available, the bridging concept morphs into open-ended treatment.

9. The American Medical Association has long held the position that direct-to-consumer advertising of pharmaceuticals should be restricted. Only recently has this position been gaining traction. But no practical restrictions really exist.

CHAPTER THREE: THE DENIAL OF OLD AGE: IMMORTAL IN AMERICA?

1. Ezekiel Emanuel, MD, is a provost at the University of Pennsylvania, an oncologist, and a bioethicist. He is a thought leader in medical ethics and end-of-life issues.

2. James Fries, MD, was a Kaiser Fellow and at Stanford University when he wrote an article entitled "Aging, Natural Death, and the Compression of Morbidity," *New England Journal of Medicine* 303, no. 3 (1980): 130–5. The concept was refined and updated in an essay in *The Milbank Quarterly* 83, no. 4 (2005): 801–23.

3. Ernst Wynder, MD, was an American epidemiologist who studied the negative health effects of tobacco smoke and wrote that "it should be the function of medicine to help people die young as late in life as possible."

4. Michael Chernow and David Cutler, Harvard academicians, have written a comprehensive review of the disability-free life expectancy of the American population after sixty-five. They defined disability as impairment in any activity of daily living (ADL) or instrumental activity of daily living. They concluded that between 1994 and 2009, the life expectancy after age sixty-five increased from 17.5 to 18.8 years. The disability-free years increased from 8.9 to 10.7, and the disabled years decreased from 8.6 to 8.1. They also concluded that the "vast bulk" of the increase in disability-free life expectancy was the result of better

treatment of acute heart attacks and strokes as well as decreased visual problems because of more widespread cataract surgery. Improvements in disability-free years associated with the other chronic illnesses were largely unchanged.

"Understanding the Improvement in Disability Free Life Expectancy in the US Elderly Population," National Bureau of Economic Research, June 2016.

5. Eileen Crimmins, PhD, has written extensively on public health issues, aging, and disability. She has most recently concluded that over the last forty years, in the general population, life expectancy has increased but that years of disability have also increased. "There are a number of indications that the baby boomer population that is now reaching old age is not seeing improvements in health similar to the older groups that went before them." She agrees, however, that for healthy people over the age of sixty-five there is a slight decrease in the proportion of disabled years, i.e., a "compression of morbidity."

Crimmins, E. et al., "Trends Over 4 Decades in Disability-Free Life Expectancy in the United States," *American Journal of Public Health* 106, no. 7 (2016): 1287–93.

6. Sigmoid volvulus is the term for a spontaneous twist in the distal colon that obstructs the intestine. Straightening the twist with a colonoscope relieves the obstruction for an unpredictable period of time—sometimes days and sometimes years.

7. The concept of activities of daily living, as a measure of functional status, was proposed by Sidney Katz in the 1950s.

Basic ADLs help to quantify the ability to bathe, dress, use the toilet, transfer from bed to chair, maintain continence, and eat. Instrumental ADLs involve shopping, cooking, cleaning, accounting, organization of medications, telephone use, and transportation. Physical therapists and occupational therapists apply values to a patient's performance status to develop rehabilitation plans.

8. Throughout this book I am encouraging you to look objectively, yet informally, at your disease and performance status. For more insight into how this can help you understand your clinical status and associated prognostic implications, a more formal Comprehensive Geriatric Assessment can be performed by most geriatricians and some hospitals with special geriatric services. In theory, they can help with a more effective care plan.

9. Leonardo Barbosa Barreto de Brito, et al., "Ability to Sit and Rise from the Floor as a Predictor of All-Cause Mortality," *European Journal of Preventive Cardiology* (2012): 1–7.

Jane Fleming et al., "Inability to Get Up after Falling, Subsequent Time on Floor, and Summoning Help: Prospective Cohort Study in People over Ninety," *British Medical Journal* (2008): 337.

10. J. Fries, "The Compression of Morbidity," *The Milbank Quarterly* 83, no. 4 (2005): 801–23.

11. When an elderly patient was referred for a screening colonoscopy, I advised them that based on my interpretation of the data, the odds that they would die of colon cancer were one in fifty if they never had a screening colonoscopy, or one in a hundred if a screening colonoscopy had been done in the last ten years. If I performed another screening colonoscopy (as expected by the referring physician), the exam would change those odds to one in a hundred or one

in two hundred, respectively. With this small benefit in mind, most elderly patients declined the exam. Of course, if they were referred for a symptom such as abdominal pain or blood in the stool, that changed the calculation, and we addressed it thoughtfully and conservatively.

CHAPTER FOUR: THE MEDIAN *IS* THE MESSAGE

1. At the time of Alfred's treatments, chemotherapy and radiation therapy were less refined than they are today, and a wide surgical excision was still slightly more curative. Most people, however, accepted the higher risk of relapse to avoid the colostomy bag that he willingly agreed to.

2. S. J. Gould, "The Median Isn't the Message," *Discover* 6 (1985): 40–2. In this essay Professor Gould notes that the survival curve (a statistical distribution) is the result of a single set of circumstances prescribed for that particular study. If a study was performed with only forty-one-year-olds, the median survival might have been longer. And, more important, he was young and healthy enough to be included in a new experimental protocol that would also have created a completely different distribution. So, in the sense that he chose different treatment, he agreed that the median of the initial studies was the message.

3. YouTube has many videos of *The Price is Right* and Plinko players.

4. At the time of that conversation, a new concept in pancreatology was developing. Pathologists were recognizing a new illness. Autoimmune pancreatitis was a benign disease that mimicked pancreatic cancer on X-rays and was mistaken for pancreatic cancer on biopsies taken during surgery. This raised the specter that some long-term survivors of what was presumed to be pancreatic cancer did not have cancer at all.

5. An example of one study documenting decreased benefit and decreased median survival in elderly patients is: H. Sorbye, et al., "Age-dependent Improvement in Median and Long-Term Survival in Unselected Population-Based Nordic Registries of Patients with Synchronous Metastatic Colorectal Cancer," *Annals of Oncology,* 24 (9) (2013): 2354–60.

6. Remember the elderly patient in chapter 2 who insisted on treatment with an immune system modulator for her late-onset ulcerative colitis. The studies supporting its use did not include many elderly patients, and its instructions carried a warning to that effect.

7. If we accept that 250,000 patients die from medical errors annually, then medical error becomes the third most common cause of death in the United States following heart disease and cancer (Martin Makary, et al., "Medical Error—The Third Leading Cause of Death in the US," *British Medical Journal* (2016): 353. Some authors suggest that as many as 400,000 patients die annually from adverse medical events, i.e., the treatment they have received.

8. In his classic article "The Hazards of Hospitalization," Dr. Elihu Schimmel first codified the risks of medical care even when everything is done correctly. The study was undertaken because the author perceived that medical knowledge was advancing so quickly and medical care was becoming so complex that even the best care, performed well, resulted in unexpected complications.

Elihu M. Schimmel, et al., "The Hazards of Hospitalization," *Annals of Internal Medicine* 60, no. 1 (1964): 100–110.

9. Jeffrey Rothschild, et al. "The Critical Care Safety Study: The Incidence and Nature of Adverse Events and Serious Medical Errors in Intensive Care," *Critical Care Medicine* 33, no. 8 (2005): 1694–1700.

10. Polypharmacy is the concept that whenever a patient uses five or more medications (prescription or over-the-counter), the number of drug–drug interactions is unpredictable and can lead to complications.

   The liver is the site of most drug metabolism. Some drugs speed up liver metabolism of other drugs. Other drugs slow down the metabolism of some drugs. Some drugs are filtered by the kidney, other drugs damage the kidney. Many drugs have unpredictable or paradoxical effects (an effect opposite from the intended and expected effect) in elderly patients.

11. Karen Kehl's "Moving toward Peace: An Analysis of the Concept of a Good Death," see endnote 5 in chapter 1, identified twelve attributes of a good death. They are repeated here in descending order of perceived importance: being in control, being comfortable, sense of closure, affirmation of the dying person's value, trust in care, recognition of impending death, beliefs honored, burden minimized, relationships optimized, appropriateness of death, leaving a legacy, and family care.

CHAPTER FIVE: HOW DIFFERENT DISEASES LEAD TO COMMON CAUSES OF DEATH

1. Depression is frequently invoked as a major problem in old age. Psychiatric research, supported and influenced by the pharmaceutical industry, reports many beneficial effects of antidepressants. Medications are frequently prescribed and, in my experience, more frequently adjusted because of their poor efficacy in this situation despite the research to the contrary.

   In general, depression can be divided into intrinsic depression, a mood disorder, and situational depression, the result of an external event such as the death of a loved one. The former is more amenable to drug therapy and the latter improves with emotional support and the passage of time.

   I think that the depression of old age is better viewed as a situational grief and better treated with support and acceptance. The temptation to treat depression in the last years of life should be resisted when the medications, which have many side effects in the elderly, are not clearly beneficial during a trial period.

2. Geriatricians include exhaustion as a symptom of frailty and the broader concept of "failure to thrive" in the elderly. One study defined frailty as a clinical syndrome of three or more of the following symptoms: self-reported exhaustion (Dad's "fatigue"), unintentional weight loss, weakness (decreased grip strength, for example), slow walking speed, and low physical activity. The prevalence of this syndrome was 7 percent in a population of patients over sixty-five years of age and participating in a cardiovascular health study.

   L. P. Fried, et al., "Frailty in Older Adults: Evidence of a Phenotype," *The Journals of Gerontology. Series A, Biological Science and Medical Science* 56(3) (2001): M146.

3. One online resource, Data 360, estimates that the average life expectancy will increase from seventy-nine to eighty-four by 2050. This is a rate of increase of 1.7 months per year. It is not the promise of dramatically prolonged life that people have come to expect. http://www.data360.org/dsg .aspx?Data_Set_Group_Id=195.

4. When bacteria get into the blood, be it from the lungs, urinary tract, bile duct, skin, or elsewhere, they release toxins with various effects. The body, in turn, activates the immune system to counter the bacterial growth and damage. Initially, the effects of this influx of bacterial invaders and host defenses are confusion, lassitude, and weakness. At this juncture antibiotics alone might reverse the process. But the cascade of damage can still spiral out of control, and the destructive mix of toxins and antitoxins leads to low blood pressure, leaky blood vessels, fluid accumulation in the lungs, kidney shutdown, poor oxygen flow to the brain, cardiac strain—and death. At this point only care in the ICU has the potential to reverse the process. Without treatment in the ICU the patient has a comparatively quiet death. The Sepsis Alliance at www.sepsis.org is trying to increase awareness of this diagnosis, particularly as it relates to young people who can be saved with early diagnosis.

5. Among the many statistics collated by the Centers for Disease Control is "10 Leading Causes of Death by Age Group." The first column is for infants younger than one year old. The next three columns group children by the ages of 1–4, 5–9, and 10–14 years. The next five columns group people by decade (e.g., ages 15–24, 25–34...up to 55–64 years of age). The final column bears the header of "65+."

   That column, clustering sixty-five-year-olds and ninety-five-year-olds, is the subject of this chapter.

6. Sherwin B. Nuland, MD, *How We Die: Reflections on Life's Final Chapter* (New York: Vintage Books, 1993).

7. The Karnofsky Performance Status score runs from 100 to 0, where 100 is "perfect" health and 0 is dead. It was developed, decades ago, to assess a cancer patient's likelihood of survival regarding the appropriateness of a proposed treatment; in the original article it was about nitrogen mustard chemotherapy for lung cancer. Now it is widely used to evaluate a patient for the appropriateness of palliative care or eligibility for hospice admission. For example, a decline of 50 percent has significantly negative prognostic implications; that, or an advanced chronic illness and a KPS of less than 60, can be used to justify hospice admission. The KPS follows:

   - 100—Normal; no complaints; no evidence of disease.
   - 90—Able to carry on normal activity; minor signs or symptoms of disease.
   - 80—Normal activity with effort; some signs or symptoms of disease.
   - 70—Cares for self; unable to carry on normal activity or to do active work.
   - 60—Requires occasional assistance but is able to care for most of their personal needs.
   - 50—Requires considerable assistance and frequent medical care.
   - 40—Disabled; requires special care and assistance.
   - 30—Severely disabled; hospital admission is indicated, although death not imminent.

- 20—Very sick; hospital admission is necessary; active supportive treatment is necessary.
- 10—Moribund; fatal processes progressing rapidly.
- 0—Dead.

   D. Karnofsky, et al., "The Use of Nitrogen Mustards in the Palliative Treatment of Carcinoma—With Particular Reference to Bronchogenic Carcinoma." *Cancer*, 1948; 1 (4): 634–56.

8. S. Katz, T. D. Down, H. R. Cash, R. C. Grotz. "Progress in the Development of the Index of ADL," *Gerontologist*, 10 (1970): 20.

CHAPTER SIX: DEATHBED SCENARIOS: HOW DOES THE END FINALLY ARRIVE?

1. The strokes might have been caused by occasional increases in his untreated hypertension, but I know from the nursing notes that his blood pressure was generally normal despite having stopped his medications three months earlier.
2. CT scan, ventilation/perfusion scan, or angiogram.
3. S. Salpeter, "Systematic Review of Noncancer Presentations with a Median Survival of 6 Months or Less," *The American Journal of Medicine* (2012): 125
4. See endnote 4 in chapter 5. The treatment of sepsis is not simply the administration of oral antibiotics. It involves aggressive ICU care using intravenous antibiotics, supportive measures (think mechanical ventilation, hemodialysis, heating and cooling blankets, cardiac medications, bladder catheters, large-bore needles in the neck and groin, and the occasional rectal tube) and immunomodulation to counteract the bacterial toxins and the patient's wayward immune response. The poor success rate when treating advanced sepsis in the elderly should be considered before subjecting a patient to this treatment, especially if they have voiced an interest in avoiding aggressive care.
5. Jeanne and Eileen Fitzpatrick introduced me to the terms of "exit opportunity" and "exit strategy" in their book *A Better Way of Dying: How to Make the Best Choices at the End of Life,* Jeanne Fitzpatrick, MD, and Eileen Fitzpatrick, JD (New York: Penguin Books, 2010).

CHAPTER SEVEN: DAD'S FINAL WEEKS

1. Dad suffered from progressive and intermittently severe itching. While he was still seeking medical care, his physicians were unable to diagnose the cause. Later, in hospice care, it was suppressed with steroids. I wondered if it was related to a systemic effect of the lymphoma, but no other evidence of lymphoma activity was identified.
2. In the world of hospice care, "active dying" begins in the last few days of life. It is associated with disturbing sounds (the "death rattle," for instance, which probably is not painful) and dreams or visions, which are thought to be comforting.

   C. W. Kerr, et al., "End-of-life Dreams and Visions: A Longitudinal Study of Hospice Patients' Experiences," *Journal of Palliative Medicine* 17(3) (2014): 296–303.

3. L. Ganzini, et al., "Nurses' Experiences with Hospice Patients Who Refuse Food and Fluids to Hasten Death," *New England Journal of Medicine* 349 (2003): 359–65. This landmark work described hospice nurses' experience with self-dehydration, including the time course of self-dehydration for more than a hundred patients.

4. In the situation described here, these tiny cracks in the vertebrae are known as compression fractures. They are not a serious threat but, like other fractures, they are very painful and slow to heal. When recognized and diagnosed as something more than simple back pain, the pain can be improved by stabilizing the spine with a percutaneous vertebroplasty—the injection of bone cement, performed as an outpatient. My father's symptoms never rose to that level.

CHAPTER EIGHT: HOW TO RECOGNIZE A TERMINAL DIAGNOSIS

1. President Nixon declared war on cancer in 1971, and every administration since then has advanced policies and programs echoing that theme. Most recently, in 2016, President Obama announced his Cancer Moonshot Initiative.

2. There are multiple staging systems for each organ-specific type of cancer. For example, colon cancer alone has been classified by the Dukes or Astler-Coller prognostic groups, anatomic staging (as described in the text), and TNM (Tumor, Node, Metastases) staging. Your doctor can describe the best classification for the particular cancer of interest to you.

3. Studies show that cancer center advertising does not highlight treatment outcomes, largely because good quality, academic, tertiary care centers all have similar outcomes. Rather, the advertisements refer vaguely to good outcomes but highlight amenities and appeal to the viewers' emotions. The dramatic rise in advertising is evidence of its efficacy in recruiting patients despite these similar outcomes.

   L. B. Vater, et al., "What Are Cancer Centers Advertising to the Public?: A Content Analysis," *Annals of Internal Medicine* 160(12) (2014): 813–20.

4. S. R. Salpeter, et al., "Systematic Review of Noncancer Presentations with a Median Survival of 6 Months or Less," *American Journal of Medicine* 125(5) (2012): 512.

5. S. R. Salpeter, et al., "Systematic Review of Cancer Presentations With a Median Survival of 6 Months or Less," *Journal of Palliative Medicine* 15(2) (2012): 175–85.

6. J. N. Temel, et al., "Early Palliative Care for Patients with Metastatic Non–Small-Cell Lung Cancer," *New England Journal of Medicine* 363 (2010):733–42.

CHAPTER NINE: THE VALUE OF YOUR PROGNOSIS

1. The disease in question was usually alcoholic hepatitis, an inflammation of the liver that was generally reversible with abstinence and nutritional support.

2. There is much written about withholding medical information. The position of the American Medical Association is that while making some accommodation to patient preferences, whenever possible, physicians should minimize

the withholding of information. "Report of the American Medical Association Council on Ethical and Judicial Affairs: Withholding Information from Patients: Rethinking the Propriety of 'Therapeutic Privilege,'" 2006.

3. N. Christakis, et al., "Extent and Determinants of Error in Doctors' Prognoses in Terminally Ill Patients: Prospective Cohort Study," *British Medical Journal* 320 (2000): 469–73.

4. At that time in Washington, DC, EMTs were not allowed to pronounce patients at the scene of an unattended death. Because she was not yet registered as a DNR patient, had they been called before the body temperature had fallen and rigor mortis had set in, the EMTs would have been required to consider CPR. At a minimum they would have had to transport her to the nearest ER to be pronounced dead by a physician.

5. UpToDate is an online subscription service for physicians that offers succinct summaries of medical topics. It is, effectively, an online medical encyclopedia that is kept current with semiannual reviews of the pertinent literature for each topic. It is written for medical personnel but it has a free "Patient Education" section that I used to educate my father about his aneurysm. The Patient Education section is written to be understood by people with a high school education ("The Basics") or a college education ("Beyond the Basics"). The discussion about aneurysm expansion and risk of rupture was in the latter category. A table of contents is found at www.uptodate.com/contents/table-of-contents/patient-information.

6. Prognostic information from Memorial Sloan-Kettering Cancer Center is found at www.mskcc.org/nomograms.

7. For more general questions ePrognosis can help with life expectancy and the risk/benefit analysis of screening tests in the elderly. See eprognosis.ucsf.edu/calculators/#/.

8. Searching for the following will take you to the Center for Medicare and Medicaid Services (CMS) site: Local Coverage Determination (LCD): Hospice Determining Terminal Status (L34538).

CHAPTER TEN: THE HARD CONVERSATION

1. Approximately one third of community-dwelling people over the age of sixty-five fall at least once per year. Half of that group falls more than twice per year, and the occurrence of falls increases with age and medications. Antidepressants have the strongest association with an increased fall risk, but cardiac medications, sedatives, and pain medications increase fall risk, too.

    Marlies R. de Jong, et al., "Drug-related Falls in Older Patients: Implicated Drugs, Consequences and Possible Prevention Strategies," *Therapeutic Advances in Drug Safety* 4(4) (2013): 147–54.

2. It can be found at med.stanford.edu/letter.html.

3. The standard of care for her referral diagnosis, iron deficiency anemia, would be a colonoscopy to exclude colon cancer and an upper endoscopy (visual exam of the upper gastrointestinal tract) to exclude cancer of the esophagus, stomach, or intestine. During these exams, there was the possibility of finding one of

several benign causes for blood loss, but excluding malignancy while finding something treatable was the paramount agenda for a woman of her age.

4. A patient can "fire" or dismiss a doctor at any time and for any reason. It is rare for a physician to dismiss a patient, but when they do, it must be done at such a time and in such a way that the patient is not abandoned. In this case, because of her unreasonable demands (she demanded that emergency treatment be delayed until I could return to the hospital—despite my arrangements to have the on call gastro-enterologist treat her), I reviewed the situation with the hospital ethics committee and found another physician willing to take on her care without interruption.

5. A gallbladder attack (acute cholecystitis) is caused when a gallstone is unable to exit the narrow neck of the gallbladder. It is associated with a bacterial infection of the biliary system. The standard of care is surgical removal of the gallbladder because that offers the possibility of a permanent solution. But, when the risk of surgery is very high because of serious heart or lung disease, a trial of antibiotics alone is considered. The hope is that the infection will respond, swelling will shrink, and bile flow will be restored if the offending stone falls back into the bladder. Future attacks are likely but might be months or years away.

6. K. A. Kehl, et al., "Moving toward Peace: An Analysis of the Concept of a Good Death," *American Journal of Hospice and Palliative Care*. For more, see endnote 5 in chapter 1 and endnote 11 in chapter 4.

CHAPTER ELEVEN: HOSPICE CARE

1. Dame Saunders was originally trained as a nurse. She developed an interest in caring for terminal patients. Recognizing the growing disconnects between sci-entific progress treating diseases and the ignored spiritual and emotional needs of patients, she went to medical school to better address this imbalance and spawned the hospice movement.

2. In 2010, more than 1.5 million Americans received home hospice services.

3. Some patients will need palliative care that requires skilled nursing. Examples of such care are intractable pain requiring infusions of morphine directly into the spinal canal or intractable seizures requiring high-dose intravenous infu-sions of anticonvulsants.

4. An example of aggressive palliative care might be the unexpected occurrence of a simple bowel obstruction in a patient in hospice care for Parkinson's disease. Surgery is rarely considered in hospice patients, but this patient faces the choice of slowly dying of a bowel obstruction, its pain only partially mitigated by high-dose opiates, "terminal sedation" (the administration of high-dose narcotics or sedatives to control intractable pain "foreseeing but not intending" that this might hasten a patient's death by respiratory depression or dehydration—see endnote 1 in chapter 12), or comparatively simple surgery to palliate the pain and relieve the obstruction.

5. In general, hospice admission does not require homebound status in the pres-ence of an active cancer or other terminal illness, but it does when the admitting diagnosis is "geriatric failure to thrive."

6. N. Christakis, et al., "Survival of Medicare Patients after Enrollment in Hos-pice Programs," *New England Journal of Medicine* 335 (1996): 172–8.

7. Palliative care is frequently linked with hospice care but it is also a stand-alone specialty that should be consulted whenever a serious illness is diagnosed, well before it is appropriate to begin end-of-life care. A palliative care team can work in parallel with other specialists (oncologists, surgeons, cardiologists, intensivists) to manage the difficult symptoms of serious illnesses. Once familiar with the medical benefits of palliative care, as they approach the end of life, patients are more likely to accept hospice care.

8. In most jurisdictions, in the event of a fall without injury, when people are unable to get themselves up from the floor, the fire department is called for lifting help. After entering hospice care, the hospice supplies lifting help.

CHAPTER TWELVE: VOLUNTARY REFUSAL OF FLUID AND FOOD

1. Terminal sedation is the administration of narcotics or other medications to control intractable symptoms (usually intractable pain) "foreseeing but not intending" that this might hasten a patient's death by respiratory depression or dehydration. Medical aid in dying (only available in six states—California, Colorado, Montana, Oregon, Vermont, Washington—and the District of Columbia) is when a patient seeks and a physician supplies a prescription for oral medication, with information on its use and the understanding that the patient might use it to end their life.

2. Again, see endnote 3 in chapter 7. L. Ganzini, et al., "Nurse's Experience with Hospice Patients Who Refuse Food and Fluids to Hasten Death," *New England Journal of Medicine* 349 (2003):359–65.

EPILOGUE: REFLECTIONS AND A ROAD MAP

1. One biologic treatment, Portrazza (necitumumab) costs $11,430 per month and extends life by six weeks (from about 38 weeks to 44 weeks). American Pharmacist's Association bulletin, December 18, 2015. Another, Opdivo (nivolumab) extends life by three months but 50 percent of patients suffer severe side effects. The cost of initial therapy is approximately $150,000 with an additional monthly cost of $14,000. Michael Wilkes, MD, PhD, U.C. Davis in *Health News Review*, December 16, 2015, at healthnewsreview.org.

2. See endnote 5 in chapter 1, Kehl, "Moving toward Peace: An Analysis of the Concept of a Good Death," *American Journal of Hospice and Palliative Care*, 2006.

3. One exception to this advice might be the patient early in the course of chronic heart failure where cardiac arrest is more likely to be from a reversible rhythm disturbance (ventricular fibrillation). In this rare circumstance limited CPR with early cardioversion is marginally more successful than the grim statistics that I have quoted elsewhere.

APPENDIX I: ADVANCE DIRECTIVES

1. Estate.findlaw.com is a site that accesses the statutes regarding advance directives in every state.

2. The health care power of attorney is distinct from the financial power of attorney, although in some cases they may be the same person or agent.

3. See endnote 3 in chapter 1 about the failure of CPR in sick or frail elderly patients. Keep in mind that almost every survivor of CPR will have broken ribs, a bruised heart, internal bleeding, and a prolonged stay in the ICU. And the rare elderly survivor is not likely to be discharged home but more likely to be discharged to a nursing home with a reduced physical and neurological capacity.

4. See endnote 3 in chapter 7. This article, "Nurses' Experience with Hospice Patients Who Refuse Food and Fluids to Hasten Death," was well researched and generally favorable in its description of declining oral intake, the characteristics of patients who chose voluntary self-dehydration, the time course of the process, and the quality of death that resulted. Therefore, I wanted my parents' living wills to reflect their appreciation of that process.

5. Example of dementia clause: My advance directive addresses my particular wishes in the event of a terminal illness and an unconscious state. This provision will specify that if I remain conscious but have a progressive illness that is likely to be fatal, is deemed irreversible, and has rendered me unable to communicate, care for myself, recognize my family, or safely swallow food or fluid (Alzheimer's disease, for example), then I want all my particular wishes to be followed as if I were unconscious.

6. Example of transfer clause: I understand that because of circumstances beyond my control I might be admitted to a health care institution whose policy is to decline to follow my Advance Directive instructions that are in conflict with its religious or moral teaching. I direct that if the health care institution in which I am a patient declines to follow my wishes as set out in my Advance Directive, then I am to be transferred in a timely manner to a hospital, nursing home, or other institution that will agree to honor my instructions.

APPENDIX II: DEMENTIA

1. Most commonly, thyroid disease, vitamin B deficiencies, heavy metal toxicities, chronic infections (e.g., syphilis and HIV-related disorders) can be mistaken for dementia. If properly diagnosed, these can be treated. Less commonly, abnormal intracranial pressure mimics dementia and sometimes responds to treatment.

2. A majority of patients over the age of sixty, hospitalized with advanced cancer, heart, or lung disease, and who had placed no limits to aggressive care, advised interviewers that they would just as soon be dead rather than have to tolerate regular incontinence or open-ended mechanical ventilation, tube feeding, or bed-bound care by others.

   Emily Rubin, et al., "States Worse Than Death Among Hospitalized Patients With Serious Illnesses," *JAMA Internal Medicine* 176(10) (2016;):1557–59.

3. The legislatures of Minnesota, New Hampshire, New York, and Wisconsin have banned the withdrawal of manual feeding.

4. Opinion 2.20—"Withholding or Withdrawing Life-Sustaining Medical Treatment," *AMA Journal of Ethics, Virtual Mentor* 15, no. 12 (2013): 1038–40.

Resource List

Please note that online resources for end-of-life decision making are infinite. The following list is, therefore, very incomplete. I have selected them simply as good, representative examples of the types of resources available. I have no connection with any of them—other than being a longtime subscriber to UpToDate.

CHAPTER FIVE: HOW DIFFERENT DISEASES LEAD TO COMMON CAUSES OF DEATH

For general information about any disease, I recommend looking at UpToDate, a for-profit, online medical encyclopedia that offers medical information to doctors and patients for a subscription fee, although a subscription can be limited to a week or a month at a time. A free patient information portal offers information at two different reading levels. **The Basics—UpToDate**, will connect you to information suitable for a reader with a fifth- to sixth-grade reading level. **Beyond the Basics—UpToDate** will link you to information for the high school and college level reader.

This type of information should be used as a starting point for discussions with your physicians.

CHAPTER EIGHT: HOW TO RECOGNIZE A TERMINAL DIAGNOSIS

In this chapter, while discussing terminal diagnoses, I have recommended seeking consultations with palliative care experts and geriatricians. Either specialist is likely to be better versed in discussing prognoses than your primary care physician. Furthermore, they will be able to manage the symptoms of aging and identify the best time for hospice care admission. The issue is how to find a good fit with a well-trained physician.

Both palliative care and geriatrics are relatively new subspecialties. Some physicians (older internists or family practitioners, for example), seeking a slower practice schedule, have rebranded their practices and relabeled themselves as geriatricians. They might be fine physicians but they are likely to bring old habits rather than the newest academic thinking to their rebranded practices. Therefore, I suggest seeking out board certified experts for palliative or geriatric care consultations.

Unfortunately, web-based services such as **Healthgrades.com** or **Vitals.com** that supply the names and ratings of physicians are highly unreliable as to character, affability, and actual ability. **HealthinAging.org**, the patient information site of the American Geriatrics Society, will give you a list of board certified geriatricians in your area, but again, there is little other reliable information.

If you get most of your care from a large, multidisciplinary medical group, it is likely to have a geriatrician or palliative care specialist on staff. If you are receiving assistance from an outpatient nursing and home health aide service, its geriatric care manager will be able to recommend such consultants. If neither of these situations describes you, and if your primary care physician is unable (or unwilling) to refer you to a board certified geriatrician or palliative care expert, I suggest you call the palliative care department of your local, trusted hospital and discuss your questions with the head nurse of the service. Seeking their insight into personalities of the local physicians will likely find you a better match than an anonymous website. Similarly, the doctors and nurses of a nearby hospice will have insight into local resources.

CHAPTER NINE: THE VALUE OF YOUR PROGNOSIS

In general, prognostic information is best interpreted with the help of your doctors— ideally your primary care physician in consultation with a geriatrician or palliative care physician.

UpToDate has limited, but useful, prognostic information.

Most academic cancer centers have diagnosis-specific prognosis algorithms. In this chapter, I used Memorial Sloan-Kettering Cancer Center (**mskcc.org**) simply as one example.

In the absence of a specific diagnosis, but in the presence of old age and frailty, **ePrognosis.ucsf.edu.org** can offer some prognostic information about life expectancy and the benefits (or lack thereof) of common screening exams.

CHAPTER TEN: THE HARD CONVERSATION

There are multiple online resources available to learn about starting The Conversation. Almost every hospice organization and end-of-life site will have advice to offer. Based on my reading and on their affiliations, I suggest looking at the following:

Theconversationproject.org, a group that works with the Institute for Healthcare Improvement to foster better end-of-life decisions through better communication, was founded by Ellen Goodman, the former newspaper columnist; **acpdecisions.org**, which offers a series of videos about advance care planning, was created by Angelo Volandes, a Harvard physician and author of *The Conversation*; and, **med.stanford.edu/letter** is a link to the Stanford Letter Project, which will help you develop your vision and communicate with your physician.

CHAPTER ELEVEN: HOSPICE CARE

The most important resources for issues related to hospice care are the National Hospice and Palliative Care Organization (**nhpco.org**) and its consumer education program, **caringinfo.org**. An alternative is the Hospice Foundation of America (**hospicefoundation.org**).

For reviewing the government's guidelines that qualify a patient for hospice coverage through Medicare or Medicaid, search **Local Coverage Determination (LCD): Hospice Determining Terminal Status (L34538)**.

CHAPTER TWELVE: VOLUNTARY REFUSAL OF FLUID AND FOOD

In looking for resources that might help you better understand the process of hastening death by voluntarily refusing to eat and drink, I became frustrated by the hidden agendas behind each site. When there was a religiously conservative perspective, self-dehydration was described as more painful than it was in my experience. When there was a liberal right-to-die bent, the dying process was generally described as too peaceful to align with my experience.

To maintain the objectivity that this important decision requires, I recommend only two resources. The first is **UpToDate**, but this will require a one-week subscription, selecting the section on "Stopping Artificial Nutrition and Hydration at the End of Life," going to the subsection "Voluntary Cessation of Intake," and working through the medical references—too much for most people. The second recommendation is your local hospice professional.

The vast majority of people considering self-dehydration as a means to hasten death are in hospice care or are candidates for hospice care. Furthermore, patients who undertake terminal dehydration need the support (emotional, medical, and pharmaceutical) of palliative care experts. Therefore, discuss this option with your primary physician first and subsequently with palliative care experts (physicians and nurses) as the decision nears.

APPENDIX I: ADVANCE DIRECTIVES

Estate.findlaw.com is a website that will help you access the statutes governing advance directives in any given state. This information is also available on the hospice sites.

POLST.org is the website of the National POLST Paradigm. This has information about POLST programs across the country.

The National Hospice and Palliative Care Organization and Compassion & Choices have websites that deal extensively with end-of-life issues. Either of their associated websites (**nhpco.org** or **compassionandchoices.org**) can help stimulate the creation of a living will.

Aging with Dignity, another nonprofit organization, is the creator of the Five Wishes program at **agingwithdignity.org**. The Five Wishes program helps you create a living will in everyday language that is a valid advance directive in the majority of states.

APPENDIX II: DEMENTIA

Again, the most important resource for the average patient with dementia will be their physicians and the recommendations that they make.

In reviewing online resources, three organizations stand out. The Alzheimer's Foundation of America (**alzfdn.org**) is a consortium that unites 2,600 member organizations. Its website is particularly good for finding local resources for all forms of Alzheimer's support and treatment. The Alzheimer's Association (**alz.org**) is a voluntary health organization leading in advocacy for Alzheimer's care, support, and research. And **Alzheimers.net** is an online community advocating for the education and support of patients and caregivers. It has a particularly interesting blog discussing caretaking trials and tribulations.

Index

Abdominal aortic aneurysm (AAA), 49–50, 85, 89–90, 136, 137, 152–53, 225
Abdominal surgery, 78, 153
Abscesses, 75, 106
Acceptance of death, xiv, xvii, 222–23
"Actively dying," 114, 118, 202, 207–9, 263*n*
Activities of daily living (ADLs), 41, 260*n*
Acute complications of chronic diseases, 18–19
Acute illnesses, 69–72
Adams, John, 40
Advance care planning, 217, 229. *See also* Advance directives
Advance directives, 229–44
  The Conversation about, 161, 162, 163–64, 171
  creating your own, 238–39
  definitions, 230–32
  dementia and, 249–51, 269*n*
  exit strategy and, 243
  father's story, 114, 159, 161
  interactions and overlapping of documents, 232–35
  limited care vs. palliation, 239–40
  oral vs. written, 242–43
  resources, 238–39, 273
  timing of, 241–42
  trying to live forever, 240–41
Adverse events, 56–57, 261*n*
Advertising, 25–26, 46–47, 259*n*, 265*n*

Aggressive passivity, xvii, 11, 109, 139, 212, 240
Aging With Dignity, 239, 273
Air mattresses, 180, 181, 186
Alcohol, 146–47
Allen, Henry "Red," 40
Allen, Woody, 119
Alzheimer's disease, 26, 80–82, 245–53
  advance care planning for, 249–51
  "buying some time" vs. natural death, 252–53
  mission creep in, 246–48
  natural death and, 251–52
  pneumonia and, 103–5
  resources, 274
  suffering caused by treating advanced, 248–49
American diet, 18–19, 34–35, 73
American exceptionalism, and momentum to treat, 24, 28–29
American health care system, xvii, 12–27
  author's confronting of medicine's limits, 19–21
  commercialization of care, 12–13, 214–15
  expenditures, 12–13, 15
  "medicalization" of death, 7–9
  momentum to treat, 23–26
  overemphasis on screening programs, 18–19
  overuse of antibiotics, 21–23
  promises vs. reality check, 213–14

American health care system (*cont.*)
  role of Medicare, 14, 24
  technology and aging, 14–16
  vision of living vs. fighting to the end, 26–28
American immortalists, xv–xvi, 29–30, 31, 35, 36
Amyotrophic lateral sclerosis (ALS), 70, 121–23
Anesthesia, 69, 78
Annual physical exams, 44–45
Antibiotic associated colitis (AAC), 23
Antibiotics, 69, 70, 181
  overuse of, 21–23, 259*n*
  sepsis and, 106–7
Antidepressants, 65, 262*n*, 266*n*
Antioxidants, 29, 33
Anxiety control, 180
Appetite loss, 66, 75, 205, 207
Arc of disease. *See* Disease trajectories
Asimov, Isaac, 196
Aspiration pneumonia, 105, 207, 246, 247
Assembly-line care, 14–17
  medical consequences of, 16–17
Assisted living, 9, 39, 217
Assisted suicide, xiii–xiv, 11, 198
Atherosclerosis, 73, 79, 83, 100
Average life expectancy, 13, 30–32, 218
  compression of morbidity, 30, 32, *32,* 43
  disabled years after sixty-five, 32–33
  gender differences, 258*n*
  healthy lifestyles and, 34–35
  increase in, 263*n*
  loss of performance status, 67–69, *68*
  medical care after seventy-five, 35–36
  survival curve, 30–31, *31, 32,* 51–53

Baby boomers, 26, 30, 33, 260*n*
"Best death," 10–11
"Better death," xvii, 9–11
  definition of, 11
Bile duct cancer, 102, 151–52
Bladder infections, 44, 90, 106
Blueberries, 35
Breast cancer, 4, 57, 58–59, 130–31, 139
Bronchitis, 76, 77

Cancer, 26, 75–76. *See also* Terminal cancer; *And specific forms of cancer*
  Patrick's case, 87–88
  plus second chronic illness, 131–33
  staging, 124, 265*n*
  war on, 26, 124, 265*n*
Cancer centers, 126, 265*n*
Cancer trials, 132
Can't We Talk about Something More Pleasant? (Chast), 168
Cardiomyopathy, 100
Caring Connections, 238
Carter, Jimmy, 119
Center for Medicare and Medicaid Services (CMS), 135
Centers for Disease Control and Prevention (CDC), 71, 72, 93, 106
Cerebrovascular disease. *See* Strokes
Chast, Roz, 168
Chemotherapy, 58, 126, 127–29, 131, 132–33
Chernow, Michael, 259–60*n*
Christakis, Nicholas, 143
Chronic illnesses, 63–64, 72–84
  cancer, 75–76
  case studies, 86–88
  chronic obstructive pulmonary disease, 76–78
  congestive heart failure, 72–75
  dementia, 80–82
  diabetes mellitus, 82–84
  old age as, 84–85
  old age as a diagnosis, 65–67
  overemphasis on screening programs, 18–19
  pattern recognition, 88–89, 92–93
  strokes, 78–80
Church, role of, 178–79
"Churning," 15
Cleveland Clinic, 24
Clostridia difficile, 22–23, 77
Colon cancer, 19–21, 35, 46, 102, 259*n*
  Alfred's story, 50–51
Colonoscopies, 19–21, 45–47, 166–67, 259*n*
Comfort care. *See* Palliative care

Comfort kits, 186–87, 188, 193
Comfort vs. cyclical treatment, 89–90
Commercialization of medical care, 12–13, 214–15
Comorbidity, 131–32
Compassion & Choices, 238–39
Competitive health care systems, 24–25
Comprehensive Geriatric Assessment, 260*n*
Compression of morbidity, 30, 32, *32, 43,* 259*n*
Congestive heart failure (CHF), 72–75, 169
  on death certificate, 99–101
  John's case, 86–87
Conversation, The, 157–76. *See also* Hard Conversation
  denial and, 158, 165–69
  father's story, 159–61
  how to start, 158
  legal perspective, 162
  moral perspective, 164–65
  resources, 272
  strategies for, 170–72
  terminal cancer and, 129
  time line for, 161–62
Coolidge, Susan, 177
COPD (chronic obstructive pulmonary disease), 76–78, 134
Council on Ethical and Judicial Affairs, 251–52
CPR (cardiopulmonary resuscitation), 7–8, 101, 163, 171, 219, 231, 257*n*
Crimmins, Eileen, 260*n*
Crowley, Candy, 245
Cutler, David, 259–60*n*

Davis, Adele, 34
Death, definitions of, 10–11
Deathbed scenarios, xvii–xviii, 92–109. *See also* Death certificates
  exit strategies, 107–9
  sepsis and, 105–7
Death by self-dehydration, 197–200. *See also* Voluntary refusal of fluid and food

Death certificates, 93–105, 115
  causes of death, 94–95
  father's, 94–96, 110
  pneumonia and, 103–5
  representative, 96–103
Death trajectory curve, 67–69, *68*
Debility, 40–41, 42–43
Dementia, 26, 80–82, 245–53
  advance care planning for, 249–51
  "buying some time" vs. natural death, 252–53
  mission creep in, 246–48
  natural death and, 251–52
  pneumonia and, 103–5
  resources, 274
  suffering caused by treating advanced, 248–49
Denial, and The Conversation, 158, 165–69
Denial of old age, 28–48
  arbitrary decisions vs. vision or plan, 47–48
  disability of old age, 40–41
  disabled years after sixty-five, 32–33
  medical care after seventy-five, 35–37
  more care vs. less care, 44–47
  quality of life after sixty-five, 41, 42–44
  statistical concept vs. lifestyle goal, 30–32
  strategy to die better, 37–38
  survival curve, 30–31, *31, 32*
Depression, 65, 66, 262*n*
Diabetes mellitus (DM), 82–84
Diet, 18–19, 29, 33, 34–35, 73
Disability of old age, 40–41
Disease prevention, and lifestyle choices, 18–19, 34–35
Disease trajectories, xiv, xvii–xviii, 63–91, 219
  acute illnesses, 69–72
  case studies, 86–88
  choosing comfort vs. cyclical treatment, 89–90
  chronic illnesses. *See* Chronic illnesses

Disease trajectories (*cont.*)
  common death trajectory curve,
    67–69, *68*
  on death certificates, 93–94
  death trajectory curve, 67–69, *68*
  old age as a chronic disease, 84–85
  old age as a diagnosis, 65–67
  pattern recognition, 88–89, 92–93
DNR (Do Not Resuscitate), 101, 217,
    231, 234–35
  definition of, 231
  dementia and, 250
  discussion with doctor, 219
  father's story, 6, 161, 183–84
  Sarah's story, 168
Durable Power of Attorney for Health
    Care, 230–31, 232–33
"Dying of old age," 135
"Dying young, late in life," 31, 33

Eisenhower, Dwight D., 12–13
Elective (or semi-elective) surgeries, 15,
    16, 17, 36, 163
Electrocardiogram (EKG), 74
Emanuel, Ezekiel J., 29–30, 37–38, 47,
    106–7, 218, 259*n*
Emergency medical technicians
    (EMTs), 7, 266*n*
Emotional acceptance of death, xiv, xvii,
    222–23
Emphysema, 76–77
End-of-life conversations. *See*
    Conversation, The; Hard
    Conversation
End-of-life prognosis, 150–53
End-of-life (exit) strategies, xiii–xiv,
    37–38, 107–9. *See also* Voluntary
    refusal of fluid and food
  advance directives and, 243
  father's story, 111–12, 200–202
  hospice care, 109, 177–95
  specific steps to take, 216–20
  visualizing quality of final days, 138–39
Endoscopies, 45–46
Endovascular aneurysm repair (EVAR),
    153

EPrognosis, 155, 266*n*, 272
Escape Fire (Nissan), 12
Euphoria, and refusal of fluid and food,
    201, 202, 204
Exercise, 29, 33, 34
Exit strategies. *See* End-of-life strategies

Falls (falling), 71, 193, 266*n*, 268*n*
Family network, 217
Fatigue of old age, 65–67, 136–37
Financial interests in medical care,
    12–14, 214–15
Financial power of attorney, 269*n*
Fixx, Jim, 34
Forgetfulness, 81–82
Frailty, 65–67, 136–37, 262*n*
Fries, James, 30–31, *31*, 43, 259*n*

Gawande, Atul, 157
Genetics (genes), 42, 76, 81
"Geriatric failure to thrive," 135
Geriatricians, consultation with, 218,
    219
"Giving up," 59, 139, 197, 220–21
"Good death," 10–11, 174
  attributes of, 175, 215–16, 262*n*
  father's story, 3–4, 6–7
  mother's story, 4–6
Gould, Stephen Jay, 51–52, 261*n*
Government policy, and life expectancy,
    32–33
Gray, John, 49

Hand-feeding, 206–7
Hard Conversation, 157–58
  denial and, 158, 165–69
  father's story, 159–61
  hope and, 172–75
  medical perspective, 163–64
  moral perspective, 164–65
  resources, 272
  time line for, 161–62
Harrington, Deborah R. (mother),
    xii–xiii, 43–44, 97
  abridged chronology of decline, 224
  acceptance of diagnosis, 222–23

"good death," 4–6
  hospice care, 183–85
  lung cancer diagnosis, 4, 6, 43, 49,
    56, 125–26, 145–46, 148
  urosepsis, 221–22
Harrington, John T. (father)
  abridged chronology of decline,
    224–26
  acceptance of death, 222–23
  antibiotic-related complications,
    21–23
  The Conversation, 159–61
  deathbed scenes and, 116–17
  death certificate, 94–96, 110
  failure to thrive, 136–37
  fatigue of old age, 65–67, 136–37
  final days, 207–9
  final moments, 115
  final weeks, 110–18
  "good death" and, 3–4, 6–7
  hospice care, 110–15, 185–88, 191
  influence of pain, 117–18, 209
  manageable death, xii–xiii, xviii,
    38–40, 49–50, 64–65, 89–90, 96,
    115, 229
  median survival, 49, 52–53
  old age as a diagnosis, 65–67
  old age as chronic disease, 84–85
  prognostic information, 152–54
  quality of life, 43–44
  refusal of fluid and food, 112,
    114–15, 197–98, 200–202, 203,
    205, 206, 207–9
  "waking up dead," 6, 8–9, 160–61
  wife's death and, 4, 5, 6, 64, 116, 136,
    160–61, 183–85
Health care systems, competition
  between, 24–25
Healthy lifestyles, 18–19, 34–35
Heart valve replacements, 73, 214
Henley, William Ernest, 52
Henson, Jim, 70–71
Hippocrates, 92
Hope and the Hard Conversation,
  172–75
Hopelessness, 59, 120, 174–75

Hospice care, 109, 177–95
  alternative medical system, 194–95
  brief history of, 178–79
  early admission, 181–82, 189, 192
  father's story, 110–15, 185–88, 191
  Medicare admission criteria, 135,
    137, 181–82
  medication list, 186–87, 219–20
  overtreatment and, 177, 188, 190, 193
  pain management, 209
  parameters of, 192–94
  as a philosophy, 179–80
  as regulatory concept, 181–82
  resources, 272–73
  terminology, 178, 183
  as treatment program, 180–81
  understanding and accepting benefits
    of, 188–92
Hospital beds, 181, 186
Hospitalists, 15–16, 258n
How We Die (Nuland), xvii–xviii, 63, 84
Hunger, 201, 202, 209
Hyponatremia, 100

Idiopathic sepsis, 106
Immortalists, xv–xvi, 29–30, 31, 35, 36
Immortalization Commission, The
  (Gray), 49
Incontinence, 22–23, 106, 108–9
Infliximab, 25–26
Influenza (flu), 71, 201
"In hospice," 179, 183
Instrumental activities of daily living
  (IADLs), 41, 260n
Insurance, 12. *See also* Medicare
  for long-term ventilatory support,
    122
Internal organs and aging, 57–58
Isaacson, Walter, xv

Jefferson, Thomas, 28, 40, 55, 57
Jenkins, Farish, 59–60
Jobs, Steve, xi, xv
Johns Hopkins Hospital, 24
Joint replacements, 15, 16, 36
Jurisdictional standards, 162, 217, 230

Karnofsky Performance Status (KPS), 85, 134, 246, 263–64n
Kaufman, Sharon, 23–24
Kehl, Karen, 215, 258, 262
Kidney failure, 71, 74, 102–3, 202
Kübler-Ross, Elizabeth, xiv

Lacunar strokes, 79, 95
Left ventricular assist device (LVAD), 24–25, 259n
Legal issues, 162, 217. *See also* Advance directives
  refusal of fluid and food, 198, 206–7, 252–53
Life expectancy, average. *See* Average life expectancy
Lifestyle choices, 18–19, 34–35
  safety concerns, 217
Liver disease, 66, 87, 102, 134, 146–47
Liver failure, 74, 96, 102–3, 146
Living wills, 230, 233–34, 242
  sample, 236–38
Local Coverage Determinants (LCDs), 156
Lou Gehrig's disease, 70, 121–23
Lung cancer, 51, 132, 139, 194, 213, 257n
  on death certificate, 96, 97–99
  mother's story, 4, 6, 43, 49, 56, 125–26, 145–46
Lung disease, 50–51, 134. *See also* COPD
  Patrick's case, 87–88
  pneumonia and, 103–5

Magical thinking, 59, 60
Mammography, 19, 130, 131
Manual feeding, 206–7
Mayo Clinic, 24, 55
Mechanical lifts, 113–14, 181, 226
Mechanical ventilation, 78, 122–23, 157
"Median Isn't the Message, The" (Gould), 51–52, 261n
Median is the message, 58–60
Median survival, 49–60, 257n
  aging and internal organs, 57–58
  aging patients and, 55–56

father's story, 49, 52–53
  medical complexity and, 56–57
  randomness and, 53–55
  survival curve, 51–53, *52,* 261n
Medical aid in dying, xiii–xiv, 196–97, 204, 210
Medical care after seventy-five, 35–37
Medical complexity, 56–57
Medical disk drop, 54
Medical errors, 56–57, 261n
Medical-industrial complex, 12–13, 26, 258n
"Medicalization" of death, 7–9
Medical passivity, xvii, 11, 109, 139, 212, 240
Medicare, 14, 24
  hospice care admission criteria, 135, 137, 181–82
Mental puzzles, 29, 33
MOLST (Medical Orders for Life Sustaining Treatment), 217, 219
Momentum to treat, 23–26, 47
  American exceptionalism and, 24, 28–29
  will to live and, 28–29
Morphine, 77, 96, 105, 114, 203
"Mother test," 46, 211–12
Muscle loss, 41, 57, 73–74
Muscle weakness, 73–74, 100

National Hospice and Palliative Care Organization, 109, 238
Nissan, Steven, 12
Nixon, Richard, 265n
Nonmalignant terminal illnesses, 133–35
NSAIDs (non-steroidal anti-inflammatory drugs), 17
Nuland, Sherwin, xvii–xviii, 63, 84
Nursing homes, 8, 9–10, 39, 157, 217
  John's story, 86–87

Obama, Barack, 265n
Old age
  as a chronic disease, 84–85
  denial of. *See* Denial of old age
  as a diagnosis, 65–67

disability of, 40–41
fatigue of, 65–67, 136–37
measurements, 85
as terminal, 135
Oncologists, 125–29, 132–33
Online resources. *See* Resources
Ordinary Medicine (Kaufman), 23–24
Osler, William, 107, 136
Overtreatment, 14, 177

Pain management, 180, 209
father's story, 117–18, 209
Palliative care, 89–90, 139, 239–40,
    267–68*n*
hospice and, 180, 190
terminal cancer and, 127–29
Pancreatic cancer, 55, 102, 116, 127,
    130, 139, 147, 155, 172–73
Paradigm shifts, 213–14
Paraneoplastic condition, 132–33
Parkinson's disease, 82, 205, 267*n*
Patient Self-Determination Act of 1991,
    163–64, 206, 251
Performance status, 218–19
father's story, 38, 40, 41
Karnofsky Performance Status, 85,
    134, 263–64*n*
loss of, 41, 67–69, *68,* 108
Pharmaceutical advertising, 25–26,
    259*n*
Philosophy of care, 179–80
Physical exams, 44–45
Physician-assisted suicide, xiii–xiv, 11,
    198
Plinko, 53–54
Pneumonia, 103–5, 106
CHF and, 74
Jim Henson's story, 70–71
Osler on, 107, 136
POLST (Physician Orders for Life
    Sustaining Treatment), 217, 219,
    231–31, 235
Polypharmacy, 58, 262*n*
Price is Right, The (TV show), 53–54
Primary care physicians, 14, 128–29,
    191, 219

Prognosis, 143–56, 218
either/or vs. along a time line,
    144–46
end-of-life, 150–53
father's story, 152–54
Old World vs. New World patients,
    149–50
researching, 154–56, 272
use of term, 145–46
when recovery is not possible, 147
when recovery is possible, 146–47
withholding information, 148–50
Promises vs. reality check, 213–14
Prostate cancer, 58, 59, 116
Prostate cancer blood tests, 19
Pulmonary edema, 100, 101
Pulmonary embolus (PE), 97–98, 104

Quality of life
after sixty-five, 42–44
vs. quantity of life, 177

Reality check, 213–14
Rectal cancer, 50, 58
Refusal of fluid and food. *See* Voluntary
    refusal of fluid and food
Rehabilitation, 41, 42, 73
Relman, Arnold, 12–13
Resources, 271–74
advance directives, 238–39, 273
researching your prognosis, 154–55,
    272
Right-to-die laws, 217, 251

Sacks, Oliver, 211
Safety call buttons, 159, 161, 176
Saunders, Cicely, 179–80, 267*n*
Schimmel, Elihu, 261*n*
Screening programs, 18–19, 46–47
Second opinions, 25, 46, 128, 151, 164
Sepsis, 105–7, 264*n*
Septicemia, 71, 72
Service lines, 15–16
Skin care, 180
Smoking, 50, 54, 55, 76, 85, 132, 259*n*
Spiritual support, 178, 184, 187, 239

Stage II cancer, 124
Stage III cancer, 124
Stage IV cancer, 124, 125, 127
Stanford Letter Project (SLP), 164, 272
Steroids, 101–2, 181
Stress reduction, 33
Strokes, 70, 78–80
  pneumonia and, 103–5
"Sundowning," 189–90
Support network, 217
Survival curve, 30–31, *31, 32,* 51–53,
  52, 261*n*
Systemic effects, 98–99, 132–33

targeted behaviors, 34–35
Technology
  aging and, 14–16, 26, 69
  screening programs and, 20
Terminal cancer, 123–33
  hospice care and, 180
  oncology, palliative care, and The
    Conversation, 127–29
  plus second chronic illness, 131–33
  Sally's story, 129–31
  standardized treatments, 126
Terminal conditions, definition of, 120
Terminal illnesses, 119–40. *See also*
  Terminal cancer
  acknowledging, 120–21
  The Conversation and, 165–69
  dealing with reality of, 121–23
  definition of, 120
  father's story, 136–37
  nonmalignant, 133–35
  old age as terminal, 135
  terminology, 120
  visualizing quality of final days,
    138–39
"Terminal," use of term, 120
Thomas, Dylan, 51–52
Transfer clause, 269*n*
Transient ischemic attacks (TIAs), 79
Treatment risks, 35–37, 56–58
Tufts University, 24–25

TV disk drop, 53–54
Type 1 diabetes, 82
Type 2 diabetes, 82–84, 86

Ulcerative colitis, 25–26, 71, 101–2, 261*n*
Unconsciousness, 94, 160
UpToDate, 153, 155, 266*n,* 273

Ventricular fibrillation, 96, 99–100, 104
Vision of death, 47–48, 49–50, 89–90,
  107–8, 138–39, 218
Vision of living, 26–28
Vitamins, 29, 34
Volandes, Angelo, 157
Voluntary refusal of fluid and food,
  196–210
  dehydration as part of natural death,
    198–200
  father's story, 112, 114–15, 197–98,
    200–202, 203, 205, 206, 207–9
  hand-feeding, 206–7
  legal implications, 198, 206–7
  length of, 204–5
  offering sense of control, 210
  physiology of, 202–4
  practical, ethical, and legal aspects,
    197–98
  resources, 273
  timing the initiation of, 205–6

"Waking up dead," 6, 8–9, 11, 160–61
Welch, H. Gilbert, 258–59*n*
"Why I Hope to Die at 75" (Emanuel),
  29–30, 37–38, 47, 106–7, 218
Wiesel, Elie, 110
Wills, 162
Will to live, xi, xv, 28–29, 51, 53, 60
Withholding medical information,
  148–50, 265–66*n*
World War II, 116–17
Wynder, Ernst, 259*n*

"You Might Get Better But You'll Never
  Get Well" (song), 40

About the Author

SAM HARRINGTON, an honors graduate of Harvard College and the University of Wisconsin Medical School, practiced internal medicine and gastroenterology for more than thirty years in Washington, DC. There he served on the board of trustees of Sibley Memorial Hospital, a member of the Johns Hopkins Health System, and the former Hospice Care of DC. He currently serves on the boards of The Island Nursing Home, a nonprofit nursing home, and Ready By 21, a mentoring program for students, both on Deer Isle, Maine.

In 2013, Sam retired from clinical practice to focus on writing and health care reform. Since then he has coauthored a blog with his wife of forty-five years titled *Gap Year After 60* and has been published in the *Washington Post*. This is his first book.

When not writing, lecturing, volunteering in his community, or traveling, Sam spends time with his six grandchildren, splits wood, and hauls lobster traps (recreationally).